Organ Preserving Approaches in the Treatment of Rectal Cancer

Organ Preserving Approaches in the Treatment of Rectal Cancer

Edited by

Ben Creavin, MD

St. Vincent's University Hospital

Dublin, Ireland

Desmond Winter, MD

St. Vincent's University Hospital

Dublin, Ireland

OXFORD

UNIVERSITY PRESS

OXFORD
UNIVERSITY PRESS

Great Clarendon Street, Oxford, OX2 6DP,
United Kingdom

Oxford University Press is a department of the University of Oxford. It furthers the University's objective of excellence in research, scholarship, and education by publishing worldwide. Oxford is a registered trade mark of Oxford University Press in the UK and in certain other countries.

Published in the United States of America by Oxford University Press
198 Madison Avenue, New York, NY 10016, United States of America.

British Library Cataloguing in Publication Data
Data available

Library of Congress Control Number: 2025947220

ISBN 978–0–19–884332–0

DOI: 10.1093/med/9780198843320.001.0001

Printed and bound by
CPI Group (UK) Ltd., Croydon, CR0 4YY

Contents

Contributors

Matthew R. Albert, MD, FACS, FASCRS
Colon and Rectal Surgery
AdventHealth Medical Group Colorectal Surgery at Orlando
Orlando, Florida, United States

Vincent Assenat, MD
Visceral and Digestive Surgeon
Clinic Tivoli
Bordeaux Colorectal Institute
Bordeaux, France

Simon Bach, BMedSci (Hons), MBBS, MD, FRCS (Gen.)
Department of Cancer and Genomic Sciences
Professor of Colorectal Surgery/Head of Section—Surgery
Clinical Lead D3B Early Phase Trials Unit, CRUK Clinical Trials Unit
Consultant Colorectal Surgeon, Queen Elizabeth Hospital Birmingham
England, United Kingdom

Ishwarya Balasubramanian, MCh, FRCSI
General Surgery
Royal College of Surgeons
Ireland

Geerard L. Beets, MD, PhD
Chair Department of Surgery
Maastricht University Medical Centre
Maastricht, Netherlands

Regina G.H. Beets-Tan, MD, PhD
Professor of Radiology
Maastricht University
The Netherlands

Pim J.W.A. Burger, MD
Oncological Surgeon
Catharina Cancer Institute
Catharina Hospital
Eindhoven, Netherlands

Maxime K. Collard, MD, PhD
Hospital Practitioner
General and Digestive Surgery Department
Saint-Antoine Hospital
Sorbonne University Faculty of Medicine
Paris, France

Ben Creavin
St. Vincent's University Hospital
Dublin, Ireland

Quentin Denost, MD, PhD
Visceral and Digestive Surgeon
Clinic Tivoli
Bordeaux Colorectal Institute
Bordeaux, France

Jesse Fischer MBChB, MMedSc, FRACS
Colorectal Surgeon and Senior Lecturer
Department of Surgery
Waikato Hospital and University of Auckland
Hamilton, New Zealand

Marc-Olivier François, MD
Visceral and Digestive Surgeon
Clinic Tivoli
Bordeaux Colorectal Institute
Bordeaux, France

Frank A. Frizelle ONZM, MBChB, MMedSc, FRACS, FACS, FASCRS, FNZMA, FAMA(hon) FRCSI(hon), FRCSEd(hon)
Professor of Surgery, Otago University
Editor-in-Chief, *New Zealand Medical Journal (NZMJ)* and *Pacific Health Dialog (PHD)*
President, Colorectal Surgical Society of Australia and New Zealand (CSSANZ)
Chair, Bowel Cancer Research, Aotearoa
Chair, Christchurch Cancer Foundation
New Zealand

James Glasbey, MBBCh, BSc, MRCS, PhD
NIHR Academic Clinical Lecturer in Global Surgery and General Surgery Registrar
University of Birmingham, England
United Kingdom

Angelita Habr-Gama, MD, PhD
Professor of Surgery (Emeritus)
University of São Paulo School of Medicine
Angelita & Joaquim Gama Institute
São Paulo, Brazil

Alexander G. Heriot, MD, MBA, FRACS
Consultant Colorectal Surgeon
Director, Cancer Surgery, Peter MacCallum Cancer Centre
Director, Lower GI Tumour Stream, Victorian Comprehensive Cancer Centre
Honorary Clinical Professor, University of Melbourne
Department of Cancer Surgery
Peter MacCallum Cancer Centre
Melbourne, Australia

Roel Hompes, MD, PhD, FASCRS(hon)
Consultant Colorectal Surgeon
Division of GI Surgery
Cancer Center Amsterdam
Amsterdam University Medical Centers
Amsterdam, Netherlands

Guilherme Pagin São Julião, MD
Colorectal Surgeon
Hospital Alemão Oswaldo Cruz
São Paulo, Brazil

Michael E. Kelly, PhD, FRCSI
Chair of Surgery—Trinity College Dublin
Trinity St. James Cancer Institute
Dublin, Ireland

Tijmen Koëter, MD, PhD
Gastrointestinal Surgeon
Department of Surgery
Elkerliek Hospital/Radboudumc
Netherlands

Miranda Kusters, MD, PhD
Colorectal Surgeon
Amsterdam UMC
Amsterdam, Netherlands

Doenja M.J. Lambregts, MD, PhD
Radiologist
Netherlands Cancer Institute
Amsterdam, Netherlands

Jérémie H. Lefèvre, MD, PhD
University Professor
Hospital Practitioner
General and Digestive Surgery Department
Saint-Antoine Hospital
Sorbonne University Faculty of Medicine
Paris, France

Andrew McCombie, PhD
Research Officer and Data Analyst
Department of General Surgery
Te Whatu Ora Waitaha (Health New Zealand Canterbury)
Christchurch, New Zealand

Brenda Murphy, MD
Consultant General/Colorectal Surgeon
Beaumont Hospital
Dublin, Ireland

Per J. Nilsson, MD, PhD
Senior Lecturer
Associate Professor of Surgery
Division of Coloproctology
Department of Pelvic Cancer
Karolinska University Hospital
Stockholm, Sweden

Barbara Noiret, MD
Visceral and Digestive Surgeon
Clinic Tivoli
Bordeaux Colorectal Institute
Bordeaux, France

Lauren O'Connell, MD, FRCSI
Advanced Colorectal Cancer Fellow
Peter MacCallum Cancer Centre
Melbourne, Australia

Cinthia Denise Ortega, MD, PhD
Abdominal Radiologist
Clinics Hospital of the Faculty of Medicine, University of São Paulo (HCFMUSP)
São Paulo, Brazil

Lloyd Pereira, PhD
Medical Scientist
Molecular Diagnostic Pathology
Peter MacCallum Cancer Centre
Victorian Comprehensive Cancer Centre
Level 4, Molecular Pathology
Melbourne, Victoria, Australia

Rodrigo Oliva Perez, MD, PhD
Director, Colorectal Surgery Division
Hospital Alemão Oswaldo Cruz
São Paulo, Brazil
Editor-in-Chief, *Techniques in Coloproctology*

Femke P. Peters, MD, PhD
Radiation-Oncologist
Department of Radiotherapy
Netherlands Cancer Institute
Amsterdam, Netherlands

Robert G. Ramsay, PhD
Honorary Professor
Research Division
Peter MacCallum Cancer Centre
Department of Clinical Pathology
The University of Melbourne
Melbourne, Australia

Harm J.T. Rutten, MD
Professor, Maastricht UMC
Surgeon Oncologist, Catharina
Hospital—Eindhoven
Netherlands

Éanna J. Ryan, MB BCh, MSc, MD, FRCSI
Centre for Colorectal Disease
St. Vincent's University Hospital
Dublin, Ireland

Kieran Sheahan
UCD Full Clinical Professor, UCD School of Medicine
Consultant Histopathologist, Pathology Department
President, International Collaboration on Cancer Reporting (ICCR)
St. Vincent's University Hospital
Dublin, Ireland

Rutger C.H. Stijns, MD, PhD
Gastrointestinal Surgeon
Catharina Hospital Eindhoven
Researcher
Radboudumc Nijmegen
Nijmegen, Netherlands

Bruna Borba Vailati, MD
Colorectal Surgeon
Hospital Alemão Oswaldo Cruz
São Paulo, Brazil

Eva L.K. Voogt, MD
Erasmus University Medical Center
Rotterdam, Netherlands

Kasmira C. Wilson, BSc(Hons), MBBS, PhD, FRACS
Sir Peter MacCallum Department of Oncology, The University of Melbourne
Division of Cancer Research/Division of Cancer Surgery, Peter MacCallum Cancer Centre
Melbourne, Australia

J.H.W. (Hans) de Wilt, MD, PhD
Professor of Surgical Oncology
Department of Surgical Oncology and Gastrointestinal Surgery
Radboud University Medical Center
Department of Surgery
Nijmegen, Netherlands

Desmond Winter
St. Vincent's University Hospital
Dublin, Ireland

Alexandra Zaborowski, MD, PhD
Centre for Colorectal Disease
St. Vincent's University Hospital
Dublin, Ireland

Jan Žmuc, MD, PhD
Surgical Oncologist
Department of Surgical Oncology
Institute of Oncology Ljubljana
Slovenia

1

History of organ preservation

Watch and wait (WW) strategy

Angelita Habr-Gama, Bruna Borba Vailati, Cinthia Denise Ortega, Guilherme Pagin São Julião, and Rodrigo Oliva Perez

Historical considerations

There are many controversies regarding the pioneer implementation of neoadjuvant radiation or chemoradiation for the treatment of rectal cancer. Different centres introduced the concept of using chemoradiation or radiation before surgery as an attempt to result in tumour downsizing and downstaging.[1,2] In some of these centres, tumour response to treatment would allow local excision as an alternative to total mesorectal excision (TME). Different forms of radiation delivery were reported to result in significant tumour regression followed by full-thickness local excision as a definitive treatment strategy.[3] However, non-operative management of these patients was exclusively considered among patients with prohibitive comorbidities and definitive refusal to surgical resection and, therefore, an exceptional management strategy.

The active search and identification of patients with clinical, endoscopic, and radiological findings consistent with a clinical complete response (cCR), regardless of medical comorbidities, or refusal to surgical resection, to be considered for no immediate surgery and strict surveillance alone, was only first reported in 1998, by the group in São Paulo headed by Prof Angelita Habr-Gama.[4] From the very beginning, the necessary pre-requisite for patients undergoing the surveillance programme was the achievement of a cCR.

A few interesting facts are worth mentioning here. First, the original data was presented at the 1998 ASCRS annual meeting in San Diego, USA—as an oral presentation. This data comprised the preliminary experience since the very first patient managed by this approach in 1991. The presentation was largely and openly criticized for the 'unacceptable' removal of surgical resection from the treatment algorithm of rectal cancer. Questions from the audience were not allowed as the moderators at the time refused to open the paper for discussion.

Second, even though the submission did reach publication in Diseases of Colon & Rectum a few months later, there was no mention to the term 'Watch & Wait' (WW).[4] Even though we commonly used this WW term in clinical practice, it was only used to refer to this treatment strategy in scientific publications years later when the concept became clear to the surgical community.[5] Third, this preliminary data reported on the outcomes of a series of patients managed by observation alone after achieving a cCR with no group for comparison. Finally, the manuscript clearly states that non-operative management of these patients was envisioned by the fact that a significant proportion of patients previously managed by nCRT followed by surgery presented pathological complete response (pCR).[4] Therefore, from the very beginning, non-operative management was an attempt to avoid potentially unnecessary surgery to these patients. This contrasts with many of the early experiences reported elsewhere, where patients were managed non-operatively exclusively due to prohibitive medical comorbidities to surgical resection or definitive refusal to surgery.

Rationale

Even though no previous experience reported the use of active non-operative management of rectal cancer, clinical observations with anal cancer clearly influenced the idea of 'watch and wait'.[6] Shortly after the implementation of multimodal therapy with chemo and radiation for squamous cell anal cancer, Norman Nigro reported on the outcomes of patients who achieved a complete clinical response undergoing potentially unnecessary surgery (inevitably being abdominal-perineal excisions). Nigro also reported on the successful oncological outcomes of patients who refused radical surgery in this setting. Therefore, the anticipation of the possibility of a pCR led Prof. Habr-Gama's group to consider routine assessment of tumour response to nCRT prior to definitive surgical or even non-surgical management of these patients. Clearly, the main reason for avoiding radical surgery here was the need for a definitive stoma. Ultimately, this seems to be a relevant expectation from patients during rectal cancer treatment.[7] However, avoiding the considerable morbidity, functional consequences, and even mortality were also seen as potential benefits of this approach.

The first studies

Oncological outcomes

In order to even be considered as a valid alternative, WW had to demonstrate that this was not compromising oncological outcomes to these patients. A series of studies were subsequently published to attest the acceptable oncological outcomes after no immediate surgery among patients who achieved a cCR after nCRT. The very first study was the game changer.[8] Patients that achieved a cCR managed by WW were compared to a control group—patients with pCR after radical surgery. If there was any benefit of radical surgery among these patients, one would expect to see this in such head-to-head comparison. However, there were no differences in overall or disease-free survival that could indicate any benefit in radical surgery in the setting of a complete response. The findings reported here were the necessary spark to fire a widespread understanding of the WW concept, potential benefits, and pending limitations.[8]

Keep your friends close and your enemies closer

Even though there was a clear change in the recognition and understanding of the concept of WW after the publication of the *Annals of Surgery* paper, there was still a general scepticism among the medical and surgical oncology community.[8,9] Multiple position statements and editorials were published highlighting the risks and drawbacks of the WW.[10,11] In order to address this, an international multidisciplinary meeting (*FICARE*®) was established in São Paulo to promote a scholarly discussion of the issues, benefits, and limitations of the implementation of WW in patients achieving a cCR after nCRT. This biennial meeting (since 2007) gathered specialists in all of the related specialties in rectal cancer management and allowed the discussion of actual clinical cases. Critics of the WW were frequently invited faculty during the meeting to thoroughly address all potential risks with the approach as well as to provide clear understanding of the strictness of the selection criteria, surveillance details, and oncological outcomes. Establishment of this scientific forum exclusively dedicated to the management of rectal cancer was instrumental to the dissemination and understanding of the concept through the following years.

Local recurrences or regrowths

One of the most significant concerns after the WW strategy was the risk of developing a local recurrence, meaning reappearance of the primary cancer within the rectal wall or at the mesorectal compartment.[12,13] Studies attempted to focus on the patterns of local recurrence and on the outcomes during salvage of these patients. Initial reports suggested that patients with initial 'apparent' cCR followed by a local recurrence were successfully salvaged by radical surgery.[13] Also, these patients had similar oncological outcomes to patients managed by 'immediate' radical surgery following nCRT completion.[5] Altogether, the data suggested that development of local regrowth would otherwise not compromise oncological outcomes of patients with initial 'apparent' cCR.

The majority of local recurrences were predominantly intraluminal (90%) and rarely exclusive mesorectal.[13] Also, the vast majority of them were amenable to salvage R0 surgery. Finally, the most relevant risk factor for its development is baseline T-status (every increase in baseline T-status seems to be associated with a 10% increase in the risk for a local recurrence).[14,15]

Finally, in order to distinguish local recurrences in the setting of an initial apparent cCR (maintaining the rectum *in situ*) from a local recurrence following TME or local excision (frequently not amenable to salvage and associated with poor oncological outcomes), an arbitrary decision to name the former clinical scenario as local regrowths instead of local recurrence was reported in 2014.[16]

Definition and standardization of cCR

While all of the studies so far reported on the achievement of a cCR using clinical, endoscopic, and radiological studies, no formal attempt was made to clearly illustrate or standardize the definition of findings consistent with a cCR. In 2010, the first pictorial description of cases with endoscopic videos was published suggesting that a whitening of the mucosa, frequent telangiectasia, and absence of ulceration of the rectal mucosa were findings consistent with cCR.[17] There was also a description of a regular mucosal surface felt by digital rectal examination (DRE) despite the presence of a firm and subtle loss of pliability of the area previously harbouring the primary cancer during endoscopic examination.

However, radiological assessment was largely inconsistent for a number of years. During the early period, endorectal ultrasound and computed tomography were used to assess disease at baseline and after initial treatment. Unfortunately, these imaging modalities were insufficient to support the achievement of cCR or to identify possible mesorectal residual disease. Fortunately, considering that 90% of local regrowths presented intraluminal disease, DRE and endoscopic studies would compensate largely for the lack of any useful radiological imaging modality in detecting incomplete responses of tumour regrowth.[13]

Magnetic resonance (MR) was not yet available at the beginning of the experience, and structured interpretation of MR images only became available after 2006 with the first series of publications from the MERCURY study group.[18,19] Quality of images provided by MR evolved over time and had a tremendous impact in the assessment of tumour response (Fig. 1.1). A clear and pictorial description of the radiological findings provided by MR during response assessment became available only after uptake of the WW by groups in Europe with high expertise in MR imaging in rectal cancer.[20,21] The identification of areas of low-signal intensity (present in multiple formats) is currently included in the synoptic reporting of MR studies in routine clinical practice to assist identification of patients likely to have achieved a cCR.[20,21] In addition, precise assessment of the mesorectal compartment provides an indispensable tool during the assessment of tumour response and surveillance of patients entering the WW pathway.[22]

From single-centre to multi-centre experience

Once the concept was clearly established and preliminary oncological experience suggested the safety of this approach, different centres began to report individual

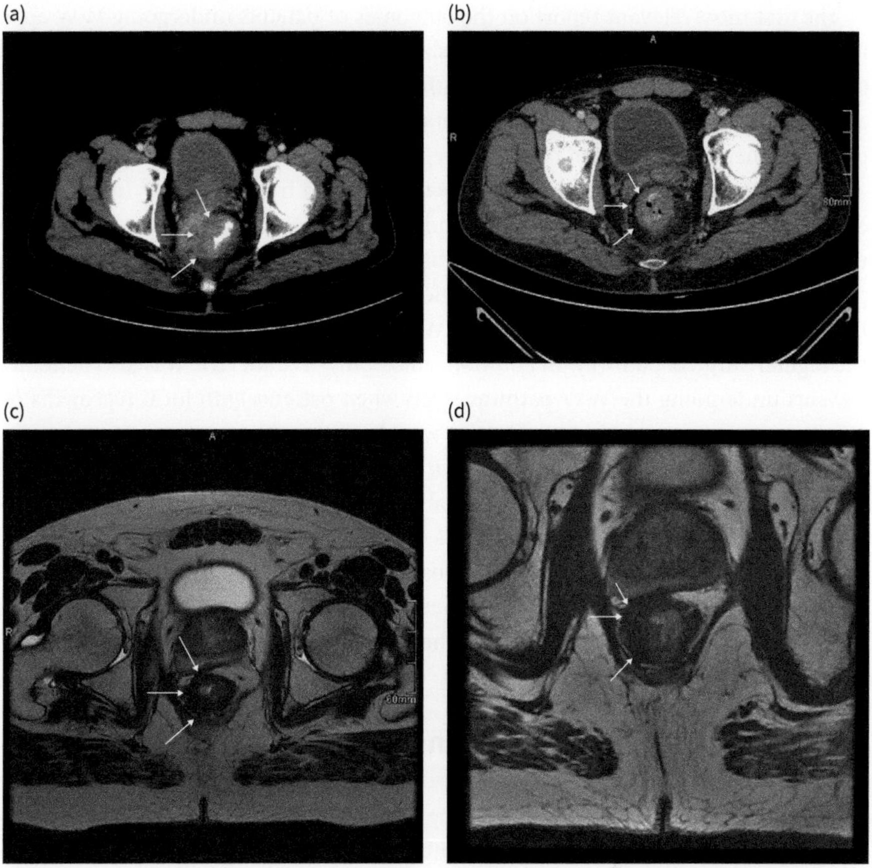

Fig. 1.1 (a) Evolution of the quality of radiological imaging of the rectum over time. Baseline assessment of a locally advanced disease (right lateral wall rectal cancer, arrows) at pelvic contrast-enhanced computed tomography (CT) with positive rectal contrast. Reassessment CT shows disappearance of lateral rectal wall thickening (b, arrows). Long-term follow-up radiological surveillance performed using magnetic resonance with a non-dedicated protocol reflected by the considerably large field of view (FOV). Low-signal intensity suggests a very good response, despite the suboptimal image definition (c, arrows) Final surveillance with MR using more contemporary parameters provided a smaller FOV leading a clear identification of the complete radiological response suggested by the presence of an area of low-signal intensity on T2-weighted image (d, arrows).

experiences with the WW strategy. Clearer definitions of findings consistent with a cCR (both endoscopic and radiological) may also have contributed to the uptake of this alternative strategy in the management of select patients undergoing nCRT. Several small case series were then reported showing similar oncological outcomes as originally reported among patients managed non-operatively.[23]

The first most relevant report on the outcomes of patients undergoing WW apart from Prof Habr-Gama's group was published by the Dutch group showing excellent oncological and functional outcomes with the WW approach.[24] The most relevant addition here was the routine implementation of MR imaging for the baseline and post-treatment assessment of response for the selection of appropriate candidates.

The second thought-provoking study was published from the UK.[25] In this multi-centre experience with WW, patients undergoing WW were compared to patients undergoing the regular surgical pathway using propensity score analysis to adjust for potentially relevant variables in oncological outcomes. While the study attempted to demonstrate the non-inferiority of WW, overall survival was actually superior to the regular surgical pathway. In addition, colostomy-free survival was also better for patients undergoing the WW pathway, even when patients with local regrowths requiring salvage were considered. The tide was clearly turning.[26]

The multiple series reported allowed for the publication of systematic reviews and meta-analyses focusing on the oncological outcomes comparing WW to radical surgery.[23] While the risk of local regrowth is expectedly higher in the WW (compared to TME where regrowth is virtually impossible after removal of the primary), non-endoluminal recurrence-free, distant metastases-free, and overall survival are all similar when comparing the two approaches.[23,27]

Changes in regimens: From nCRT towards TNT

The vast majority of patients entering the WW pathway included patients who received a long-course chemoradiation (5FU-based chemo).[28] The proportion of patients who ultimately achieve a cCR has been a matter of controversy for a long time. Even though baseline staging may affect the chances of achieving a cCR, changes in neoadjuvant treatment regimens have been extensively investigated to allow for any significant increase in the chances of a complete response. Initial studies attempted to incorporate additional chemotherapy agents into chemoradiation regimens (in addition to 5FU). However, additional chemotherapy agents (namely oxaliplatin) resulted only in increased toxicity without the expected benefit in increased pCR or cCR rates.[29]

In 2006, Prof Habr-Gama's group proposed the use of additional chemotherapy cycles during the resting period immediately after radiation completion.[30] Even though the concept was not established at that time, this was the first attempt to use consolidation chemotherapy with the specific aim to increase complete response rates. Concomitantly, consolidation chemotherapy (using 5FU exclusively) patients were treated by slightly higher doses of radiation for the same purpose. Initial reports using nCRT with consolidation chemotherapy led to an increase in the proportion of patients achieving a cCR.[31] These findings were confirmed by a non-randomized trial where patients were offered nCRT followed by progressively higher number of mFOLFOX cycles following nCRT completion. Even though cCR rates were not reported, pCR rates were significantly higher among patients receiving higher number of mFOLFOX cycles.[32]

More recently, the concept of total neoadjuvant therapy in rectal cancer became popular for two specific purposes: first, advancing delivery of adjuvant chemotherapy to treat upfront potential micrometastatic disease; second, increasing the chances of a complete response—suggested by initial experiences in the USA. In this setting, TNT would allow two different approaches: (1) chemotherapy alone followed by nCRT (induction chemotherapy); (2) nCRT followed by chemotherapy alone (consolidation chemotherapy).[33] A preliminary report on the outcomes of the OPRA trial comparing these two approaches for the purpose of achieving a cCR suggested that consolidation CRT is associated with a higher chance of achieving a cCR and entering WW when compared to induction CRT.[34]

While short-course radiation therapy followed by consolidation chemotherapy has been reported from the RAPIDO trial to result in high rates of pCR, there is still no data to support that pCR rates would translate into cCR rates. Future studies may be warranted to compare long-course and short-course RT in the setting of consolidation chemotherapy for this specific purpose.[35]

Accidental versus intentional WW

During the early experience with WW, patients who actually entered this pathway included cases where nCRT was required primarily for oncological purposes. This means that most (if not all) patients underwent nCRT and, eventually, by accident or by chance achieved a cCR. Achievement of a cCR was not the primary purpose of nCRT. However, a specific subgroup of patients with early-stage disease (mrT2N0) located at the level of (or very close) the anorectal ring has been considered for this treatment strategy (with nCRT). Here, patients who otherwise would not require nCRT for oncological reasons and who, until recently, were not contemplated in international rectal cancer management guidelines could benefit from the achievement of a cCR and avoiding TME. Considering the different regimens available, the modern paradox in rectal cancer was established: should we consider more aggressive treatment regimens with consolidation chemotherapy, particularly among patients with early stage disease—that would otherwise not even be considered to nCRT? Recent reports suggest that these patients considered for 'intentional' WW (early stage disease) are more likely to achieve a cCR and avoid TME when treated with more aggressive regimens.[36]

Initial versus Sustained cCR

In the very early studies of WW, cCR was only considered among patients who achieved and sustained a cCR for one year after the last day of RT.[8,17] The reason for this arbitrary time limit was the fact that, in most cases, it may take a significant amount of time for patients to achieve all clinical, endoscopic, and radiological criteria consistent with a cCR.[37] Therefore, most of the patients do not achieve all the strict criteria at the same time; and usually not at the first assessment of tumour response.[38]

However, the surgical oncology community felt that the message to the readership would be clearer if any patient not operated on after the first assessment of response was considered a cCR.[13] This means that any residual disease detected at the subsequent assessments of response (after the very first assessment of response). This led to an increase in the risk of local regrowths that are particularly detected within the first year of follow-up (even if a cCR has never been achieved but persistent residual disease is finally confirmed). This is particularly important when looking at local regrowth rates at three years of nearly 30%.[39] The majority of regrowths are detected within the first year.[27] When conditional survival is used to estimate local regrowth rates, patients who achieve a cCR and sustain it for over 1 year, the risk of subsequent local regrowth is ≤10%. Ultimately, achieving and sustaining a cCR for a period of time may be the most relevant biological information provided by these rectal cancers overriding other risk factors for local regrowth (including baseline T-status).[40]

Molecular biology in WW

After nearly 30 years of WW, several studies using molecular biology techniques have attempted to refine the selection of patients to add an additional tool to clinical assessment, endoscopy, and radiology. Several studies focused on the prediction of tumour response to nCRT using gene expression profiles, specific gene mutations, and microRNA expression levels.[41,42] Unfortunately, all of these strategies have been largely unsuccessful for two reasons: intertumoural and intratumoural heterogeneity.[42,43] Significant differences in genetic profiles of tumours between patients (intertumoural) and the presence of significantly different subpopulations of cancer cells within individual tumours (intratumoural) may have accounted for the inability to predict response based on pre-treatment biopsy samples. Future studies using cancer cell cultures in tumouroids/animal models are being investigated to test sensitivity and correlate with clinical outcomes.[44] In addition, understanding of molecular pathways may provide to new insights and the use of additional radiation therapy sensitizers in the future.[45,46]

Back to the future

Organ preservation in rectal cancer is currently at centre stage. Watch and wait is actually already included in international guidelines.[47] While the readership may think that this was an easy task, the ones who have witnessed this long journey will agree that it was not always an easy one. The idea of omitting surgery in the management of rectal cancer was a disruptive one and initially violently opposed. Angelita had to overcome common resistances and preconceptions from the past, still observed at present in many places, particularly in the surgical field and forums.[48] Importantly, the idea of organ preservation was always clearly patient-driven and patient-oriented. After being nearly ridiculed in her first report sharing the concept and initial data, some recent reports may suggest that organ preservation is almost self-evident and obvious. However, the journey is far more relevant and interesting than the destination itself. It may be uncertain whether we will ever reach a final destination in organ preservation. Still, the contributions ignited by this disruptive idea have clearly benefited innumerable patients around the globe with a significant impact on their lives. Hopefully, future improvements in neoadjuvant regimens, imaging modalities and molecular biology tools will allow the opportunity for organ preservation to a larger proportion of patients and to be implemented in a larger number of centres around the globe.

References

1. Mohiuddin M, Marks GJ. High dose preoperative radiation and sphincter preservation in the treatment of rectal cancer. *Int J Radiat Oncol Biol Phys*. 1987;13(6):839–42.
2. Stearns MW, Jr., Berg JW, Deddish MR. Preoperative irradiation of cancer of the rectum. *Dis Colon Rectum*. 1961;4:403–8.
3. Gerard JP, Chapet O, Nemoz C, et al. Improved sphincter preservation in low rectal cancer with high-dose preoperative radiotherapy: the lyon R96–02 randomized trial. *J Clin Oncol*. 2004;22(12):2404–9.
4. Habr-Gama A, de Souza PM, Ribeiro U, Jr., et al. Low rectal cancer: impact of radiation and chemotherapy on surgical treatment. *Dis Colon Rectum*. 1998;41(9):1087–96.
5. Habr-Gama A, Perez RO, Proscurshim I, et al. Interval between surgery and neoadjuvant chemoradiation therapy for distal rectal cancer: does delayed surgery have an impact on outcome? *Int J Radiat Oncol Biol Phys*. 2008;71(4):1181–8.
6. Nigro ND, Vaitkevicius VK, Considine B, Jr. Combined therapy for cancer of the anal canal: a preliminary report. *Dis Colon Rectum*. 1974;17(3):354–6.
7. Wrenn SM, Cepeda-Benito A, Ramos-Valadez DI, Cataldo PA. Patient perceptions and quality of life after colon and rectal surgery: what do patients really want? *Dis Colon Rectum*. 2018;61(8):971–8.
8. Habr-Gama A, Perez RO, Nadalin W, et al. Operative versus nonoperative treatment for stage 0 distal rectal cancer following chemoradiation therapy: long-term results. *Ann Surg*. 2004;240(4):711–17; discussion 717–18.
9. Glynne-Jones R, Wallace M, Livingstone JI, Meyrick-Thomas J. Complete clinical response after preoperative chemoradiation in rectal cancer: is a 'wait and see' policy justified? *Dis Colon Rectum*. 2008;51(1):10–19; discussion 19–20.
10. Borstlap WAA, van Oostendorp SE, Klaver CEL, et al. Organ preservation in rectal cancer: a synopsis of current guidelines. *Colorectal Dis*. 2017;doi:10.1111/codi.13960.
11. Ouaissi M, Alves A, Panis Y. Cancer infiltrant du rectum traite par radiochimiotherapie 'neoadjuvante': peut-on se passer de la proctectomie? [Invasive rectal cancer treated by 'neoadjuvant' radiochemotherapy: can we avoid rectal resection?]. *Ann Chir*. 2006;131(3):175–6.

12. Habr-Gama A, Perez RO, Proscurshim I, et al. Patterns of failure and survival for nonoperative treatment of stage c0 distal rectal cancer following neoadjuvant chemoradiation therapy. *J Gastrointest Surg*. 2006;10(10):1319–28; discussion 1328–9.
13. Habr-Gama A, Gama-Rodrigues J, Sao Juliao GP, et al. Local recurrence after complete clinical response and watch and wait in rectal cancer after neoadjuvant chemoradiation: impact of salvage therapy on local disease control. *Int J Radiat Oncol Biol Phys*. 2014;88(4):822–8.
14. Habr-Gama A, São Julião GP, Gama-Rodrigues J, et al. Baseline T classification predicts early tumor regrowth after nonoperative management in distal rectal cancer after extended neoadjuvant chemoradiation and initial complete clinical response. *Dis Colon Rectum*. 2017;60(6):586–94.
15. Habr-Gama A, Sao Juliao GP, Vailati BB, et al. Organ preservation among patients with clinically node-positive rectal cancer: is it really more dangerous? *Dis Colon Rectum*. 2019;62(6):675–83.
16. Heald RJ, Beets G, Carvalho C. Report from a consensus meeting: response to chemoradiotherapy in rectal cancer—predictor of cure and a crucial new choice for the patient: on behalf of the Champalimaud 2014 Faculty for 'Rectal cancer: when NOT to operate'. *Colorectal Dis*. 2014;16(5):334–7.
17. Habr-Gama A, Perez RO, Wynn G, Marks J, Kessler H, Gama-Rodrigues J. Complete clinical response after neoadjuvant chemoradiation therapy for distal rectal cancer: characterization of clinical and endoscopic findings for standardization. *Dis Colon Rectum*. 2010;53(12):1692–8.
18. Group MS. Diagnostic accuracy of preoperative magnetic resonance imaging in predicting curative resection of rectal cancer: prospective observational study. *BMJ*. 2006;333(7572):779.
19. Taylor FG, Quirke P, Heald RJ, et al. Preoperative high-resolution magnetic resonance imaging can identify good prognosis stage I, II, and III rectal cancer best managed by surgery alone: a prospective, multicenter, European study. *Ann Surg*. 2011;253(4):711–19.
20. Lambregts DM, Maas M, Bakers FC, et al. Long-term follow-up features on rectal MRI during a wait-and-see approach after a clinical complete response in patients with rectal cancer treated with chemoradiotherapy. *Dis Colon Rectum*. 2011;54(12):1521–8.
21. Lambregts DM, Vandecaveye V, Barbaro B, et al. Diffusion-weighted MRI for selection of complete responders after chemoradiation for locally advanced rectal cancer: a multicenter study. *Ann Surg Oncol*. 2011;18(8):2224–31.
22. Ortega CD, Perez RO. Role of magnetic resonance imaging in organ-preserving strategies for the management of patients with rectal cancer. *Insights Imaging*. 2019;10(1):59.
23. Dossa F, Chesney TR, Acuna SA, Baxter NN. A watch-and-wait approach for locally advanced rectal cancer after a clinical complete response following neoadjuvant chemoradiation: a systematic review and meta-analysis. *Lancet Gastroenterol Hepatol*. 2017;2(7):501–13.
24. Maas M, Beets-Tan RG, Lambregts DM, et al. Wait-and-see policy for clinical complete responders after chemoradiation for rectal cancer. *J Clin Oncol*. 2011;29(35):4633–40.
25. Renehan AG, Malcomson L, Emsley R, et al. Watch-and-wait approach versus surgical resection after chemoradiotherapy for patients with rectal cancer (the OnCoRe project): a propensity-score matched cohort analysis. *Lancet Oncol*. 2016;17(2):174–83.
26. Perez RO. Complete clinical response in rectal cancer: a turning tide. *Lancet Oncol*. 2016;17(2):125–6.
27. Dattani M, Heald RJ, Goussous G, et al. Oncological and survival outcomes in watch and wait patients with a clinical complete response after neoadjuvant chemoradiotherapy for rectal cancer: a systematic review and pooled analysis. *Ann Surg*. 2018;268(6):955–67.

28. Sanghera P, Wong DW, McConkey CC, Geh JI, Hartley A. Chemoradiotherapy for rectal cancer: an updated analysis of factors affecting pathological response. *Clin Oncol (R Coll Radiol)*. 2008;20(2):176–83.
29. Cancer, Leukemia Group B, Ryan DP, et al. Phase I/II study of preoperative oxaliplatin, fluorouracil, and external-beam radiation therapy in patients with locally advanced rectal cancer: Cancer and Leukemia Group B 89901. *J Clin Oncol*. 2006;24(16):2557–62.
30. Habr-Gama A, Perez RO, Sabbaga J, Nadalin W, Sao Juliao GP, Gama-Rodrigues J. Increasing the rates of complete response to neoadjuvant chemoradiotherapy for distal rectal cancer: results of a prospective study using additional chemotherapy during the resting period. *Dis Colon Rectum*. 2009;52(12):1927–34.
31. Habr-Gama A, Sabbaga J, Gama-Rodrigues J, et al. Watch and wait approach following extended neoadjuvant chemoradiation for distal rectal cancer: are we getting closer to anal cancer management? *Dis Colon Rectum*. 2013;56(10):1109–17.
32. Garcia-Aguilar J, Chow OS, Smith DD, et al. Effect of adding mFOLFOX6 after neoadjuvant chemoradiation in locally advanced rectal cancer: a multicentre, phase 2 trial. *Lancet Oncol*. 2015;16(8):957–66.
33. Cercek A, Roxburgh CSD, Strombom P, et al. Adoption of total neoadjuvant therapy for locally advanced rectal cancer. *JAMA Oncol*. 2018;4(6):e180071.
34. Garcia-Aguilar J, Patil S, Kim JK, et al. Organ preservation in patients with rectal adenocarcinoma treated with total neoadjuvant therapy. *J Clin Oncol*. 2022;40(23):2546–56.
35. Bahadoer RR, Dijkstra EA, van Etten B, et al. Short-course radiotherapy followed by chemotherapy before total mesorectal excision (TME) versus preoperative chemoradiotherapy, TME, and optional adjuvant chemotherapy in locally advanced rectal cancer (RAPIDO): a randomised, open-label, phase 3 trial. *Lancet Oncol*. 2021;22(1):29–42.
36. Habr-Gama A, Sao Juliao GP, Vailati BB, et al. Organ preservation in cT2N0 rectal cancer after neoadjuvant chemoradiation therapy: the impact of radiation therapy dose-escalation and consolidation chemotherapy. *Ann Surg*. 2019;269(1):102–7.
37. Habr-Gama A, Sao Juliao GP, Fernandez LM, et al. Achieving a complete clinical response after neoadjuvant chemoradiation that does not require surgical resection: it may take longer than you think! *Dis Colon Rectum*. 2019;62(7):802–8.
38. Hupkens BJP, Maas M, Martens MH, et al. Organ preservation in rectal cancer after chemoradiation: should we extend the observation period in patients with a clinical near-complete response? *Ann Surg Oncol*. 2018;25(1):197–203.
39. van der Valk MJM, Hilling DE, Bastiaannet E, et al. Long-term outcomes of clinical complete responders after neoadjuvant treatment for rectal cancer in the International Watch & Wait Database (IWWD): an international multicentre registry study. *Lancet*. 2018;391(10139):2537–45.
40. Sao Juliao GP, Karagkounis G, Fernandez LM, et al. Conditional survival in patients with rectal cancer and complete clinical response managed by watch and wait after chemoradiation: recurrence risk over time. *Ann Surg*. 2020;272(1):138–44.
41. Lopes-Ramos C, Koyama FC, Habr-Gama A, et al. Comprehensive evaluation of the effectiveness of gene expression signatures to predict complete response to neoadjuvant chemoradiotherapy and guide surgical intervention in rectal cancer. *Cancer Genet*. 2015;208(6):319–26.
42. Perez RO, Habr-Gama A, Sao Juliao GP, et al. Should we give up the search for a clinically useful gene signature for the prediction of response of rectal cancer to neoadjuvant chemoradiation? *Dis Colon Rectum*. 2016;59(9):895–7.
43. Bettoni F, Masotti C, Habr-Gama A, et al. Intratumoral genetic heterogeneity in rectal cancer: are single biopsies representative of the entirety of the tumor? *Ann Surg*. 2017;265(1):e4–e6.

44. Ganesh K, Wu C, O'Rourke KP, et al. A rectal cancer organoid platform to study individual responses to chemoradiation. *Nat Med.* 2019;25(10):1607–14.
45. Koyama FC, Lopes Ramos CM, Ledesma F, et al. Effect of Akt activation and experimental pharmacological inhibition on responses to neoadjuvant chemoradiotherapy in rectal cancer. *Br J Surg.* 2018;105(2):e192–e203.
46. Fernandes JM, Jandrey EHF, Koyama FC, et al. Metformin as an alternative radiosensitizing agent to 5-fluorouracil during neoadjuvant treatment for rectal cancer. *Dis Colon Rectum.* 2020;63(7):918–26.
47. Glynne-Jones R, Wyrwicz L, Tiret E, et al. Rectal cancer: ESMO clinical practice guidelines for diagnosis, treatment and follow-up. *Ann Oncol.* 2018;29(Supplement_4):iv263.
48. Habr-Gama A. Not taking 'no' for an answer. *Dis Colon Rectum.* 2018;61(1):8–13.

2

Radiological assessment of response to neoadjuvant chemoradiotherapy for locally advanced rectal cancer

Doenja M.J. Lambregts, Femke P. Peters, and Regina G.H. Beets-Tan

Role of anatomical MRI

MRI has established itself as one of the key imaging modalities for primary staging of rectal cancer. The main strengths of anatomical (mainly T2-weighted) MRI are that it offers an excellent high-contrast soft tissue resolution, combined with a relatively large field of view to allow detailed morphological assessment of the rectal wall together with the mesorectal compartment and surrounding pelvic organs and structures. This makes MRI an invaluable technique to define the T-stage (complemented by endorectal ultrasound for small superficial T1-2 tumours), N-stage and to assess the depth of tumour invasion into the perirectal fat and into important anatomical landmarks including the mesorectal fascia, anal sphincter, and pelvic organs. In the restaging setting, the diagnostic performance of MRI is limited by its inability to reliably discern remaining tumour foci within areas of radiation-induced fibrosis. As a result of successful (chemo)radiotherapy (CRT), tumours typically undergo a fibrotic transformation which can be identified by a vast decrease in signal of the tumour bed on T2-weighted MRI (see Fig. 2.1). Within this fibrosis, it can be very difficult to discriminate small areas of vital residual tumour. This impacts negatively on the diagnostic accuracy of MRI post-treatment with reported overall accuracies of 43–60% for yT-restaging as well as relatively poor interobserver agreement with kappa's in the range of 0.33–0.64.[1–4] Anatomical MRI experiences particular difficulties in differentiating patients who have undergone a complete tumour response (yT0) from patients with residual tumour. In a meta-analysis by van der Paardt et al., sensitivity to differentiate between yT0 and yT1–4 disease after CRT was only 19% (based on the results of 20 studies), indicating that most complete responders are overstaged with anatomical MRI.[5] Some studies use the MRI tumour regression grade (mrTRG) as a method to assess response to neoadjuvant treatment on anatomical MRI. The mrTRG is a five-point grading system to classify the degree of fibrotic transformation post-CRT on T2-weighted MRI and is derived from similar systems used for histopathological staging.[6] The mrTRG has been shown (mainly by research groups from the UK) to be beneficial to discriminate between good and poor response groups and to predict survival outcomes.[7,8] However, in a recent meta-analysis by Jang et al., a summary sensitivity of only 32.3% was reported for mrTRG to detect complete responders, indicating that it falls short as a tool to select patients for W&W.[9]

Role of diffusion-weighted MRI

Diffusion-weighted imaging (DWI) is a type of functional imaging modality that can nowadays easily be added to most modern scanners to any clinical MRI protocol with only a few minutes extra scan time and without the need for the injection of intravenous contrast agents. DWI bases its contrast on differences in the random movement ('diffusion') of water molecules between tissues of varying cellular density. In healthy (normocellular) tissues, there is ample extracellular tissue space in which water molecules can move relatively freely, i.e. unrestricted. This unrestricted diffusion causes a loss of signal when applying diffusion-sensitizing gradients to a T2-weighted sequence. Most solid cancers, including rectal cancer, are hypercellular in comparison with normal tissue which will lead to restricted extracellular diffusion of water and a retained high signal on diffusion-weighted images. This causes malignant lesions to stand out as high signal lesions on DWI compared to the suppressed background signal of the normal anatomy. Several reports have shown that in the restaging setting, visual evaluation of DWI as an addition to standard MRI leads to a significant improvement in diagnostic performance to differentiate patients with residual tumour within the fibrotically changed tumour bed from patients with a complete tumour response (see Fig. 2.1). Reported areas under the curve (AUCs) for MRI+DWI are in the range of 0.79-0.94 compared to AUCs of 0.67–0.81 for standard MRI only.[10–13] The use of DWI in this specific setting is therefore now recommended in the consensus guidelines on rectal MRI published by the European Society of Gastrointestinal and Abdominal Radiology (ESGAR) (14). An example of an MRI protocol including DWI used at our unit is provided in Table 2.1. So far, there is no evidence that DWI is beneficial to further determine the yT-stage in case of suspected residual tumour. A recent study by Fornell-Perez et al. found no clear benefit for DWI over standard MRI in this setting.[15]

In addition to visual evaluation, DWI can also render quantitative biomarkers that can be used to monitor response. The most well-known quantitative DWI parameter is the 'apparent diffusion coefficient' (ADC), which is inversely related to tissue cellular density. Results of studies focusing on ADC for rectal tumour response assessment have recently been summarized in a review paper by Schurink et al.[10] Prior to treatment, tumours typically show low ADC values. After treatment, ADC values

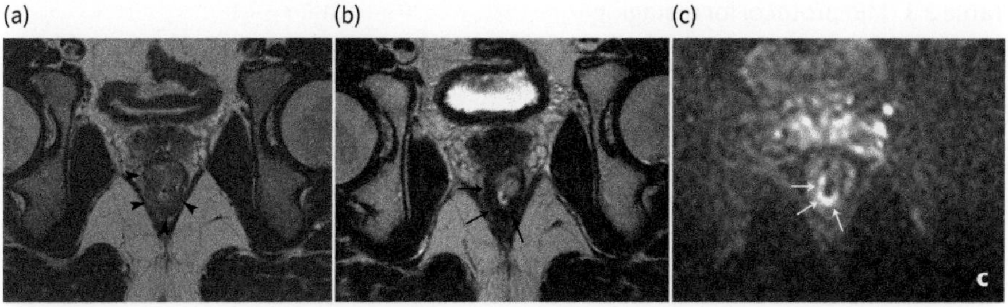

Fig. 2.1 Axial T2-weighted MRI before treatment (a) with corresponding T2-weighted (b) and b1,000 diffusion-weighted (c) MR images acquired 8 weeks after completion of chemoradiotherapy. This male patient initially presented with a semi-circular cT3b tumour in the distal rectum (black arrowheads in (a). Eight weeks after completion of CRT, the tumour shows a good response; it has decreased in volume and undergone fibrotic changes. The post-CRT T2-weighted images show a homogeneous hypointense wall thickening, indicative of fibrosis (black arrows in b). No clear solid tumour remnant is visualized. Within the fibrosis it is not possible to tell whether there are still small areas of vital residual tumour left. The diffusion-weighted images, however, still show a clear rim of high signal within the fibrotically changed tumour bed (white arrows in c), indicative of residual tumour. Histopathology confirmed a ypT2 tumour remnant. This example shows how the addition of DWI can help improve the performance of MRI to discriminate between a complete response and residual tumour in cases of fibrosis.

rise due to radiation-induced cell damage and necrosis which disrupt the presence of cell membranes resulting in increased room for extracellular water diffusion. At baseline (before treatment), ADC has been reported by some groups to correlate with the chance of successful response. High baseline ADCs have been shown to have a negative association with response, which is believed to be related to the presence of intratumoural necrosis (making tumours less susceptible to treatment effects). In addition, it has been suggested by some authors that early changes in ADC after the first weeks of radiation treatment may help to predict response. Although there is thus some evidence that ADC could act as a potential early biomarker to predict response, these positive results have been contradicted by a similar number of other research groups and the role of ADC in this setting to date remains undefined.[10] Variations in ADC between centres caused by differences in MRI hardware and methods of image acquisition and analysis will likely have also contributed to the inconsistent results in current literature. Steps towards standardization should therefore be undertaken before quantitative imaging parameters such as ADC can be implemented into clinics. Apart from ADC, some groups have also shown good results for DWI-based tumour volumetry to assess response. AUCs ranging between 0.84–0.93 have been reported to diagnose complete responders after CRT, results significantly better than for T2W-volumetry.[16–19]

Table 2.1 MRI protocol for restaging*

Field strength and hardware	• 1.5 T or 3.0 T MRI machine • External surface coil

Patient preparation	• Not mandatory
	• Optional:
	  • Spasmolytics to reduce bowel movement artefacts (particularly in high rectal tumours)
	  • A preparatory micro-enema is beneficial to reduce the amount of gas in the rectal lumen in order to avoid gas-induced susceptibility artefacts on DWI# (used routinely at our institution for restaging)

MRI sequences	• Mandatory: 2D T2-weighted (fast or turbo spin echo) sequences with a maximum slice thickness of 3 mm in at least two planes (sagittal and axial, i.e. perpendicular to the tumour axis). Optional: third coronal plane (parallel to tumour axis). • Mandatory: Diffusion-weighted imaging (DWI) sequence with at least one high b-value of ≥800 s/mm^2 (at our institution we use two b-values of b0 and b1000 s/mm^2). • Mandatory: apparent diffusion coefficient (ADC) map; to be viewed visually alongside T2W and DWI sequences. • Optional: T1-weighted sequence with a large field of view for assessment of lymph nodes and coincidental findings. • Fat-suppressed or (dynamic) contrast-enhanced sequences are not routinely recommended.

* For detailed recommendations, see ESGAR consensus guidelines on MRI for the clinical management of rectal cancer[14]

A publication by van Griethuysen et al. showed (in a cohort including a total of 335 rectal MRIs) that a preparatory micro-enema reduced the presence of significant DWI-artefacts from ± 24% to less than 4%, thereby significantly improving the diagnostic image quality of DWI.[50]

Role of other functional MRI techniques

To date, dynamic contrast enhanced (DCE) or 'perfusion' MRI is the second most widely studied functional MRI technique for response assessment in rectal cancer. DCE-MRI measures the inflow of intravenously administered gadolinium agents into tumour vessels and their leakage into the extracellular space to assess the (micro) vascular physiology of tumours. This can either be analysed semi-quantitatively, by plotting the intensity of signal enhancement after contrast injection over time, or quantitatively using pharmacokinetic models. The latter approach is more commonly used and can render quantifiable parameters of inflow and permeability, such as the Ktrans (volume rate constant, measure of vessel permeability), Ve (volume of extracellular space) and Kep (constant of flow rate). These parameters can be used as biomarkers to study angiogenesis, a known key factor associated with tumour response and prognosis. So far, most encouraging results have been reported for Ktrans as a predictor of response.[20] Ktrans values typically decrease as a result of successful treatment which is believed to be related to the replacement of vital tumour by fibrosis and necrosis. It has been shown that a lower post-CRT Ktrans is associated with a better response outcome.[20,21] Moreover, Ktrans pre-treatment tends to be higher in tumours that will show a better response to CRT and may thus have potential as a pre-treatment predictor of response.[22,23] This higher Ktrans in responders could be explained by the fact that a higher Ktrans is typically seen in tumours that show a higher vessel permeability. These tumours will typically be more susceptible to chemotherapy and tend to be better oxygenated, which in turn increases their radiosensitivity. Although common in prostate and breast cancer, more visual (qualitative) methods of response evaluation using DCE-MRI have scarcely been reported in rectal cancer. A recent report by Gollub et al. found no significant benefit for visual evaluation of DCE-MRI when added to standard MRI + DWI evaluation and endoscopy.[24]

Apart from DCE-MRI (and DWI), there are several other functional MRI techniques that have the potential to capture biological tumour properties such as oxygenation or tumour metabolism. Magnetization transfer (MT) imaging may be used to evaluate the concentration of macromolecules, including collagen, which may be beneficial to quantify the degree of fibrosis.[25] Tissue oxygenation can be indirectly measured using blood oxygenation level-dependent (BOLD) MRI. MR spectroscopy (MRS) allows the quantification of metabolic tumour changes. Evidence for these more experimental techniques is, however, limited.

In summary, there is increasing evidence that quantitative parameters derived from functional MRI have promise to act as imaging biomarkers of response, with the largest body of evidence to date existing for ADC (see previous section) and perfusion-parameters derived from DCE-MRI. For now, however, use of these quantitative parameters should be limited to the research domain. Image acquisition and analysis protocols will have to be standardized, and reproducible threshold values need to be established. Finally, large-scale multicentre validation of the predictive power of imaging biomarkers is urgently needed, preferably within the scope of clinical trials, before any of them can be implemented into routine clinical practice. To date, the only established role for functional MRI in clinics—as discussed earlier—is the visual assessment of DWI as an adjunct to standard MRI to help identify complete responders.

Role of endorectal US, CT, and PET

Endorectal ultrasound (EUS) is a well-established technique for the primary assessment of early stage, superficial tumours since it is the only technique that can provide detailed anatomical information on tumour ingrowth in the individual layers of the bowel wall, allowing for accurate distinction between T1 and T2 tumours, which is more difficult to assess with MRI. The use of EUS in the restaging setting has been less extensively studied. Overall, the reported sensitivity of EUS to identify patients with a complete tumour response after CRT is limited, ranging between 33% and 63%.[26,27] Like MRI, EUS experiences difficulties in the assessment of fibrosis, resulting in mainly overstaging errors. Because of its limited soft tissue contrast, there is no role for computed tomography (CT) in the restaging of rectal cancer. Studies that have reported on the use of CT to discriminate patients with a complete response after CRT have shown very poor results.[28–30] Positron emission tomography (PET), nowadays typically combined with CT, is not commonly used in daily clinics for the local restaging of rectal cancer after neoadjuvant treatment, despite the fact that PET/CT, in particular 18F-Fluorodeoxyglucose (FDG)-PET/CT, has been quite extensively studied for response evaluation. The commonly observed treatment effect on PET is a drop in FDG uptake after CRT caused by a decrease in tumour metabolism. This effect can be assessed visually or measured quantitatively as the standardized uptake value (SUV) or the Response Index (RI; the relative decrease in SUV compared to pre-treatment SUV) after CRT. Two separate meta-analyses reported similar pooled sensitivities of 74–78% and specificities of 64–67% to discriminate poor vs. good responding patients after CRT.[31,32] For the specific selection of complete responders, the reported performance of PET is relatively poor.[29] A study by Janssen et al. showed that only 17% of the patients with a complete metabolic remission on PET post-CRT had an actual complete response at histopathology.[33] Interestingly, the performance of FDG-PET to predict response is better when PET is performed early after the onset of radiotherapy (e.g. after 1 or 2 weeks of CRT), rather than after its completion. The meta-analysis by Li et al. reported a 10% higher sensitivity and 15% higher specificity to predict a complete response when PET was performed during rather than after CRT.[31] After treatment, false positive FDG uptake may occur due to radiation-induced inflammation, while at the same time small tumour remnants are missed owing to the relatively low resolution of PET. This limits the use of PET as a selection tool for organ preservation. In summary, PET may mainly have potential as an early predictor of response, which in the future may aid in creating opportunities for more adapted neoadjuvant treatment strategies based on the anticipated treatment response.

Lymph node response assessment

Whether patients are eligible to undergo organ-preserving treatment not only depends on the response of the primary tumour in the bowel wall, but also on the response of the lymph nodes in the mesorectum. With a watch-and-wait approach or local excision, the lymph nodes are left *in situ*. If not all nodes are sterilized, these nodes are thus a potential source for recurrence and for further dissemination. Patients with a good or complete response of their primary tumour still have a 5–16% risk of persistent nodal disease.[34] It is well-known that imaging (MRI as well as CT and EUS) has significant limitations in the primary staging of lymph nodes pre-treatment. No reliable size cut-offs exist and even with additional morphological criteria such as the nodal shape, border, and signal irregularity, nodal staging results remain insufficient.[14] Interestingly, more favourable results have been reported for nodal restaging. After CRT, the vast majority of lymph nodes decrease in size or disappear. The small nodes that remain visible have been sterilized in over 80% of the cases.[35] Nodes that remain relatively large in size after CRT are thus more likely to be malignant. These effects explain why size criteria render higher accuracies post-CRT than in the primary staging setting, albeit still with considerable variation in accuracy numbers (67–90%) in published reports.[36] Although no evidence-based size cut-offs exist, the ESGAR MRI guidelines now recommend a practical cut-off of 5 mm for nodal restaging after CRT.[4]

Lymph node-specific contrast agents such as ultrasmall superparamagnetic iron oxides (USPIOs) and gadofosveset trisodium have shown promise for nodal staging in previous studies,[37,38] but have so far not been approved for nodal staging and hence not found their way to clinical practice. Diffusion-weighted MRI is a valuable technique to detect lymph nodes due to the intrinsic high cellular density of lymphoid tissue. The downside of DWI is that both malignant, as well as benign lymph nodes will show a similarly high signal on DWI. DWI can therefore significantly increase the number of detected lymph nodes on MRI but is not accurate to discriminate between benign and malignant lymph nodes.[39] Van Heeswijk et al. reported that the visual absence of nodes on DWI after CRT renders a high sensitivity to identify yN0 patients. However, specificity was very low, since both yN0 and yN+ patients still showed high signal nodes on DWI at restaging.[40] All in all, the role of DWI for nodal restaging appears to be limited.

Timing of imaging and combination with clinical examination and endoscopy

Traditionally—before the introduction of organ preservation—surgery was performed ±6 weeks after neoadjuvant CRT, and restaging was considered optional. Nowadays, most expert centres recommend evaluating the response with longer intervals between CRT and surgery ranging between 8–10 weeks. This is related to the increasing evidence that the rate of complete responders increases with longer waiting intervals,[41,42] without evident negative effects on oncological outcome and surgical complications.[43] There is to date no clear consensus on what is the best timing after completion of neoadjuvant treatment to perform a restaging MRI. In recent literature where MRI was used to select patients for organ preservation, waiting intervals of ±8 weeks after completion of CRT were often employed.[44,45] When shorter radiotherapy schemes are used (i.e. 5×5 Gy), the difference in treatment duration should also be taken into account when assessing the response. The shorter treatment duration will typically result in less regression than with the standard five-week CRT regimen when response is assessed at the same time point, that is after the completion of treatment. To minimize the confounding effect of the various time durations of different radiation treatment schedules, it may therefore be better to define the interval considering the time point from the start of radiotherapy rather than the end of it.

The decision to opt for organ preservation is generally not based on imaging only. In 2010, Habr-Gama et al. was the first to describe the features of a clinical complete response at digital rectal examination (DRE) and endoscopy.[46] A later study by Maas et al. from 2015 showed that endoscopy is more accurate than standard anatomical MRI and also more accurate than MRI including DWI to detect complete responders, but that the best performance is achieved by combining DRE, endoscopy and MRI+DWI. This combination rendered a post-test probability of 98% to identify complete responders, versus 75% for DWI-MRI and 90% for clinical assessment (DRE and endoscopy), respectively.[47] Data from the international watch-and-wait database (IWWD), a large international multicentre registry study, showed that in 64% of the 880 registered patients a combination of MRI and endoscopy was used, indicating that this strategy is to date the most widely adopted.[48] A recent study by Haak et al. showed that MRI on its own may be a useful tool to make a first gross distinction between patients with poor response who will require surgical resection and for whom organ preserving treatment is unsafe and those with good response who may benefit from further response evaluation adding DRE and endoscopy to MRI to assess their eligibility for organ preservation.[49] Such an approach could allow more selective use of diagnostic tools.

Conclusions

The diagnostic process of assessing response in the era of organ preservation is rapidly evolving. Detailed assessment of response after neoadjuvant treatment, including the identification of patients who have undergone a complete response and may be considered for watch and wait, is now an increasingly relevant issue. Anatomical imaging techniques (MRI, EUS, and CT) are insufficiently accurate for the identification of complete responders because of difficulties in discerning viable tumour remnants within post-radiation fibrosis. The addition of functional imaging, specifically DWI, can significantly improve the performance of MRI to identify complete responders. Best results are obtained when the findings of MRI, including DWI, are combined with DRE and endoscopy. There is no clear role for PET in identifying complete responders after CRT, although PET may be valuable to predict early during treatment which patients are likely to develop a good response. Other, more quantitative functional MRI parameters derived from techniques such as DWI and DCE-MRI are emerging as potential biomarkers of response, but their value for response evaluation will need to be further established by future research. The imaging community should focus on standardization of these techniques and large-scale validation through clinical trials in order to take the next important steps towards potential clinical integration.

References

1. Kulkarni T, Gollins S, Maw A, Hobson P, Byrne R, Widdowson D. Magnetic resonance imaging in rectal cancer downstaged using neoadjuvant chemoradiation: accuracy of prediction of tumour stage and circumferential resection margin status. *Colorectal Dis.* 2008;10(5):479–89.
2. Allen SD, Padhani AR, Dzik-Jurasz AS, Glynne-Jones R. Rectal carcinoma: MRI with histologic correlation before and after chemoradiation therapy. *AJR Am J Roentgenol.* 2007;188(2):442–51.
3. Dresen RC, Beets GL, Rutten HJ, et al. Locally advanced rectal cancer: MR imaging for restaging after neoadjuvant radiation therapy with concomitant chemotherapy. Part I. Are we able to predict tumor confined to the rectal wall? *Radiology.* 2009;252(1):71–80.
4. Kuo LJ, Chern MC, Tsou MH, et al. Interpretation of magnetic resonance imaging for locally advanced rectal carcinoma after preoperative chemoradiation therapy. *Dis Colon Rectum.* 2005;48(1):23–8.
5. van der Paardt MP, Zagers MB, Beets-Tan RG, Stoker J, Bipat S. Patients who undergo preoperative chemoradiotherapy for locally advanced rectal cancer restaged by using diagnostic MR imaging: a systematic review and meta-analysis. *Radiology.* 2013;269(1):101–12.
6. Mandard AM, Dalibard F, Mandard JC, et al. Pathologic assessment of tumor regression after preoperative chemoradiotherapy of esophageal carcinoma. Clinicopathologic correlations. *Cancer.* 1994;73(11):2680–6.
7. Patel UB, Taylor F, Blomqvist L, et al. Magnetic resonance imaging-detected tumor response for locally advanced rectal cancer predicts survival outcomes: MERCURY experience. *J Clin Oncol.* 2011;29(28):3753–60.
8. Patel UB, Brown G, Rutten H, et al. Comparison of magnetic resonance imaging and histopathological response to chemoradiotherapy in locally advanced rectal cancer. *Ann Surg Oncol.* 2012;19(9):2842–52.
9. Jang JK, Choi SH, Park SH, et al. MR tumor regression grade for pathological complete response in rectal cancer post neoadjuvant chemoradiotherapy: a systematic review and meta-analysis for accuracy. *Eur Radiol.* 2020;30(4):2312–23.
10. Schurink NW, Lambregts DMJ, Beets-Tan RGH. Diffusion-weighted imaging in rectal cancer: current applications and future perspectives. *Br J Radiol.* 2019;92(1096):20180655.
11. Kim SH, Lee JM, Hong SH, et al. Locally advanced rectal cancer: added value of diffusion-weighted MR imaging in the evaluation of tumor response to neoadjuvant chemo- and radiation therapy. *Radiology.* 2009;253(1):116–25.
12. Lambregts DM, Vandecaveye V, Barbaro B, et al. Diffusion-weighted MRI for selection of complete responders after chemoradiation for locally advanced rectal cancer: a multicenter study. *Ann Surg Oncol.* 2011;18(8):2224–31.
13. Sassen S, de Booij M, Sosef M, et al. Locally advanced rectal cancer: is diffusion weighted MRI helpful for the identification of complete responders (ypT0N0) after neoadjuvant chemoradiation therapy? *Eur Radiol.* 2013;23(12):3440–9.
14. Beets-Tan RGH, Lambregts DMJ, Maas M, et al. Magnetic resonance imaging for clinical management of rectal cancer: updated recommendations from the 2016 European Society of Gastrointestinal and Abdominal Radiology (ESGAR) consensus meeting. *Eur Radiol.* 2018;28(4):1465–75.
15. Fornell-Perez R, Perez-Alonso E, Porcel-de-Peralta G, et al. Primary and post-chemoradiotherapy staging using MRI in rectal cancer: the role of diffusion imaging in the assessment of perirectal infiltration. *Abdom Radiol.* 2019;44(11):3674–82.

16. Curvo-Semedo L, Lambregts DM, Maas M, et al. Rectal cancer: assessment of complete response to preoperative combined radiation therapy with chemotherapy--conventional MR volumetry versus diffusion-weighted MR imaging. *Radiology*. 2011;260(3):734–43.
17. Ha HI, Kim AY, Yu CS, Park SH, Ha HK. Locally advanced rectal cancer: diffusion-weighted MR tumour volumetry and the apparent diffusion coefficient for evaluating complete remission after preoperative chemoradiation therapy. *Eur Radiol*. 2013;23(12):3345–53.
18. Sathyakumar K, Chandramohan A, Masih D, Jesudasan MR, Pulimood A, Eapen A. Best MRI predictors of complete response to neoadjuvant chemoradiation in locally advanced rectal cancer. *Br J Radiol*. 2016;89(1060):20150328.
19. Lambregts DMJ, Rao S-X, Sassen S, et al. MRI and diffusion-weighted MRI volumetry for identification of complete tumour responders after preoperative chemoradiotherapy in patients with rectal cancer: a bi-institutional validation study. *Ann Surg*. 2015;262(6):1034–9.
20. Dijkhoff RAP, Beets-Tan RGH, Lambregts DMJ, Beets GL, Maas M. Value of DCE-MRI for staging and response evaluation in rectal cancer: a systematic review. *Eur J Radiol*. 2017;95:155–68.
21. Intven M, Reerink O, Philippens ME. Dynamic contrast enhanced MR imaging for rectal cancer response assessment after neo-adjuvant chemoradiation. *J Magn Reson Imaging*. 2015;41(6):1646–53.
22. Tong T, Sun Y, Gollub MJ, et al. Dynamic contrast-enhanced MRI: Use in predicting pathological complete response to neoadjuvant chemoradiation in locally advanced rectal cancer. *J Magn Reson Imaging*. 2015;42(3):673–80.
23. Lim JS, Kim D, Baek SE, et al. Perfusion MRI for the prediction of treatment response after preoperative chemoradiotherapy in locally advanced rectal cancer. *Eur Radiol*. 2012;22(8):1693–700.
24. Gollub MJ, Blazic I, Felder S, et al. Value of adding dynamic contrast-enhanced MRI visual assessment to conventional MRI and clinical assessment in the diagnosis of complete tumour response to chemoradiotherapy for rectal cancer. *Eur Radiol*. 2019;29(3):1104–13.
25. Martens MH, Lambregts DM, Papanikolaou N, et al. Magnetization transfer ratio: a potential biomarker for the assessment of postradiation fibrosis in patients with rectal cancer. *Invest Radiol*. 2014;49(1):29–34.
26. Vanagunas A, Lin DE, Stryker SJ. Accuracy of endoscopic ultrasound for restaging rectal cancer following neoadjuvant chemoradiation therapy. *Am J Gastroenterol*. 2004;99(1):109–12.
27. Dickman R, Kundel Y, Levy-Drummer R, et al. Restaging locally advanced rectal cancer by different imaging modalities after preoperative chemoradiation: a comparative study. *Radiat Oncol*. 2013;8:278.
28. Huh JW, Park YA, Jung EJ, Lee KY, Sohn SK. Accuracy of endorectal ultrasonography and computed tomography for restaging rectal cancer after preoperative chemoradiation. *J Am Coll Surg*. 2008;207(1):7–12.
29. Guillem JG, Ruby JA, Leibold T, et al. Neither FDG-PET Nor CT can distinguish between a pathological complete response and an incomplete response after neoadjuvant chemoradiation in locally advanced rectal cancer: a prospective study. *Ann Surg*. 2013;258(2):289–95.
30. Jung S, Parajuli A, Yu CS, et al. Sensitivity of various evaluating modalities for predicting a pathologic complete response after preoperative chemoradiation therapy for locally advanced rectal cancer. *Ann Coloproctol*. 2019;35(5):275–81.
31. Li C, Lan X, Yuan H, Feng H, Xia X, Zhang Y. 18F-FDG PET predicts pathological response to preoperative chemoradiotherapy in patients with primary rectal cancer: a meta-analysis. *Ann Nucl Med*. 2014;28(5):436–46.

32. Zhang C, Tong J, Sun X, Liu J, Wang Y, Huang G. 18F-FDG-PET evaluation of treatment response to neo-adjuvant therapy in patients with locally advanced rectal cancer: a meta-analysis. *Int J Cancer*. 2012;131(11):2604–11.
33. Janssen MH, Ollers MC, Riedl RG, et al. Accurate prediction of pathological rectal tumor response after two weeks of preoperative radiochemotherapy using (18)F-fluorodeoxyglucose-positron emission tomography-computed tomography imaging. *Int J Radiat Oncol Biol Phys*. 2010;77(2):392–9.
34. Peeters K, Beets G, Valentini V, et al. The incidence of nodal involvement after chemoradiation for locally advanced rectal cancer: who might benefit from local excision? Results from a pooled analysis of 2386 patients. Poster presentation at ASCRS Conference, 2012.
35. Koh DM, Chau I, Tait D, Wotherspoon A, Cunningham D, Brown G. Evaluating mesorectal lymph nodes in rectal cancer before and after neoadjuvant chemoradiation using thin-section T2-weighted magnetic resonance imaging. *Int J Radiat Oncol Biol Phys*. 2008;71(2):456–61.
36. Heijnen LA, Maas M, Beets-Tan RG, et al. Nodal staging in rectal cancer: why is restaging after chemoradiation more accurate than primary nodal staging? *Int J Colorectal Dis*. 2016;31(6):1157–62.
37. Koh DM, Brown G, Collins DJ. Nanoparticles in rectal cancer imaging. *Cancer Biomark*. 2009;5(2):89–98.
38. Lambregts DM, Beets GL, Maas M, et al. Accuracy of gadofosveset-enhanced MRI for nodal staging and restaging in rectal cancer. *Ann Surg*. 2011;253(3):539–45.
39. Lambregts DM, Maas M, Riedl RG, et al. Value of ADC measurements for nodal staging after chemoradiation in locally advanced rectal cancer-a per lesion validation study. *Eur Radiol*. 2011;21(2):265–73.
40. van Heeswijk MM, Lambregts DM, Palm WM, et al. DWI for assessment of rectal cancer nodes after chemoradiotherapy: is the absence of nodes at DWI proof of a negative nodal status? *AJR Am J Roentgenol*. 2017;208(3):W79–W84.
41. Sloothaak DA, Geijsen DE, van Leersum NJ, et al. Optimal time interval between neoadjuvant chemoradiotherapy and surgery for rectal cancer. *Br J Surg*. 2013;100(7):933–9.
42. West MA, Dimitrov BD, Moyses HE, et al. Timing of surgery following neoadjuvant chemoradiotherapy in locally advanced rectal cancer—a comparison of magnetic resonance imaging at two time points and histopathological responses. *Eur J Surg Oncol*. 2016;42(9):1350–8.
43. Petrelli F, Sgroi G, Sarti E, Barni S. Increasing the interval between neoadjuvant chemoradiotherapy and surgery in rectal cancer: a meta-analysis of published studies. *Ann Surg*. 2016;263(3):458–64.
44. Martens MH, Maas M, Heijnen LA, et al. Long-term outcome of an organ preservation program after neoadjuvant treatment for rectal cancer. *J Natl Cancer Inst*. 2016;108(12):djw171.
45. Habr-Gama A, Gama-Rodrigues J, Sao Juliao GP, et al. Local recurrence after complete clinical response and watch and wait in rectal cancer after neoadjuvant chemoradiation: impact of salvage therapy on local disease control. *Int J Radiat Oncol Biol Phys*. 2014;88(4):822–8.
46. Habr-Gama A, Perez RO, Wynn G, Marks J, Kessler H, Gama-Rodrigues J. Complete clinical response after neoadjuvant chemoradiation therapy for distal rectal cancer: characterization of clinical and endoscopic findings for standardization. *Dis Colon Rectum*. 2010;53(12):1692–8.
47. Maas M, Lambregts DM, Nelemans PJ, et al. Assessment of clinical complete response after chemoradiation for rectal cancer with digital rectal examination, endoscopy, and MRI: selection for organ-saving treatment. *Ann Surg Oncol*. 2015;22(12):3873–80.

48. van der Valk MJM, Hilling DE, Bastiaannet E, et al. Long-term outcomes of clinical complete responders after neoadjuvant treatment for rectal cancer in the International Watch & Wait Database (IWWD): an international multicentre registry study. *Lancet.* 2018;391(10139):2537–45.
49. Haak H, Maas M, MJ L, et al. Selection of patients for organ preservation after chemoradiotherapy: MRI identifies poor responders who can go straight for surgery. Ann Surg Oncol. 2020;27(8):2732–9.
50. van Griethuysen J, Bus E, Hauptmann M, et al. Gas- induced susceptibility artefacts on diffusion-weighted MRI of the rectum at 1.5T—effect of applying a micro-enema to improve image quality. *Eur J Radiol.* 2018;99:131–7.

3

Radiotherapy strategies and complete response rates in locally advanced rectal cancer

Per J. Nilsson

Introduction

Treatment recommendation for an individual patient with rectal cancer should be discussed by a multidisciplinary team (MDT), and the strategy recommended depends on the stage of disease, tumour extent and patient characteristics.[1] Radiotherapy (RT) is primarily administered to reduce the rate of locoregional recurrence, but secondary aims of neoadjuvant (chemo)radiotherapy can be to achieve downsizing or downstaging whereby resectability and proportion of sphincter-saving procedures may be increased. Early tumours without adverse features are often treated with surgery alone. Locally advanced rectal cancers, e.g. with involvement of the mesorectal fascia or other organs, are usually treated with chemoradiotherapy (CRT) prior to surgery. For intermediate or locally advanced rectal cancer without threatened resection margins, either short-course radiotherapy (SCRT) or CRT before surgery is recommended. However, the preferred regimen varies between countries and institutions.[2,3] For patients at high risk of locoregional recurrence and metastatic disease, combining SCRT and some cycles of combination chemotherapy is an option.[1]

After the completion of CRT or SCRT (with delayed surgery) re-assessment of the tumour with magnetic resonance imaging (MRI) is performed. Treatment response, often expressed as tumour regression grade (TRG), is commonly reported in a four-tier scale. The optimal time period between termination of neoadjuvant therapy and re-assessment is unknown. Generally, re-assessment is recommended after 6–8 weeks, and in the Stockholm III trial restaging was performed 4–6 weeks after SCRT with delayed surgery.[4] Surgery is most often performed within 2–4 weeks after radiological re-assessment.

To obtain a clinical complete response (cCR) has not been the primary objective when delivering (chemo)radiotherapy according to these recommendations outlined briefly above. However, pathological complete response (pCR) has been observed in a proportion of rectal cancer patients in several randomized trials (Table 3.1). Obviously, a hypothetical opportunity to detect a cCR occurred among these patients

Table 3.1 Randomized trials on neoadjuvant therapy for rectal cancer

Trial	Year	Treatment groups (n)	T-stages	ypCR (%)	Ref
LARCs	2008	25×2 Gy (109)	cT3–T4	7	5
		25×2 Gy + postop chemo (98)		16	
Stockholm III	2019	5×5 Gy immediate surgery (118)	cT1–T4	0	6
		5×5 Gy delayed surgery (120)		10	
		25×2 Gy delayed surgery (65)		2	
ACCORD 12/0405	2010	25×1.8 Gy CRT Cap (282)	cT2–T4	14	7
		25×1.8 Gy CRT Capox (283)		19	
STAR-01	2011	28×1.8 Gy CRT FU (379)	cT3–T4	16	8
		28×1.8 Gy CRT FU/OX (368)		16	
CAO/ARO/AIO-04	2012	28×1.8 Gy CRT FU (606)	cT3–T4	13	9
		28×1.8 Gy CRT FU/LV/OX (591)		17	
TROG 01.04	2012	5×5 Gy immediate surgery + postop FU (162)	cT3	1	10
		28×1.8 Gy CRT FU + postop FU (161)		15	
NSABP R-04	2014	25×1.8 Gy + boost CRT Cap or FU (636)	cT3–T4	18	11
		25×1.8 Gy + boost CRT FU/OX or Capox (640)		20	
Polish Trial	2016	5×5 Gy + FOLFOX4 x3 (261)	cT3–T4	16	12
		28×1.8 Gy CRT FU/OX (254)		12	
GRECCAR 6	2016	25×2 Gy CRT Capox 7 w delay (125)	cT3–T4	15	13
		25×2 Gy CRT Capox 11 w delay (128)		17	

ypCR, pathological complete response; CRT, chemoradiotherapy; Cap, capecitabine; Capox, capecitabin/oxaliplatin; FU, 5-fluorouracil; OX, oxaliplatin; LV, leucovorin with a pCR. Thus, although patients are treated according to existing guidelines, a proportion may be offered an organ preservation strategy.

Habr-Gama and colleagues introduced the organ-sparing watch and wait strategy after cCR, including salvage surgery for patients with regrowth of tumour.[14] Since then, several reports have shown that this approach is feasible after chemoradiotherapy in prospective protocols with a 2-year regrowth rate of 16–25% and no detrimental effect on survival.[15,16]

In this chapter, published outcome data for different RT strategies and techniques are reviewed.

Long-course chemoradiotherapy

Globally, the most commonly used preoperative regimen for rectal cancer is conventionally fractionated long-course radiotherapy with concomitant chemotherapy (CRT). Radiotherapy is delivered in fractions of 1.8–2 Gy to a total dose of approximately 50 Gy, in 25–28 fractions. Chemotherapy generally consists of 5-fluorouracil (5-FU), which can be administered either intravenously or orally as capecitabine, and studies have shown equipoise between these two options. Orally administered 5-FU is logistically advantageous and may be perceived as less demanding for the patient. Chemotherapy doses administered concomitantly with CRT are somewhat lower, and total treatment time is significantly shorter, compared to when 5-FU is delivered in the postoperative adjuvant setting. Thus, the purpose of 5-FU during CRT is mainly to act as a radiosensitizer, and the systemic effect on occult metastases is limited.

CRT for rectal cancer is delivered with the aim of reducing the risk of locoregional recurrence and, in some cases, to achieve downsizing and/or downstaging. In patients with tumour extension to other organs or to the pelvic side wall (T4b), CRT increases the chance of performing a radical (R0) resection and in patients with an involved or threatened mesorectal fascia, CRT reduces the risk of local recurrence. Delivering CRT preoperatively reduces the rate of locoregional recurrence and has less toxicity compared to postoperative CRT and is therefore the standard of care.[17] Also, CRT improves local control compared to long-course RT without concomitant chemotherapy.[18] Following improvements in surgery and with a risk-stratified use of CRT, local recurrence rates of about 5% can be achieved on a national level.[19]

Although not the primary aim of CRT, pCR is obtained in a considerable proportion of patients following CRT and surgery (Table 3.1). Among patients with clinical stage T2–4 who received CRT, 12–20% had no detectable tumour in the specimen.

With the aim of improving treatment outcome and the advent of organ preserving strategies, modifications to the conventional CRT regimen have been introduced. Routes that have been explored include the addition of oxaliplatin[7–9,11] and the use of boost radiotherapy or an integrated boost.[11] In addition, the use of antibodies during

CRT has been reported.[20] The addition of oxaliplatin did not improve locoregional failure rates or survival, but toxicity was increased,[11] however, the German CAO/ARO/AIO-94 trial found that oxaliplatin added to CRT and adjuvant chemotherapy improved disease-free survival from 71.2% to 75.9%.[9] Oxaliplatin has also been investigated as induction chemotherapy before CRT and found to be feasible.[21] This regimen was explored further in the EXPERT-C trial with addition of the EGFR inhibitor cetuximab, and although response rates were improved, the primary endpoint of increased complete response was not met (9% vs. 11%, n.s.) and toxicity was more frequent.[20] The general impression is that while increased response rates can be obtained with intensified treatment the toxicity is also increased and overall survival is not affected.

An interesting Danish trial investigated high-dose CRT followed by watchful waiting as a non-operative approach.[22] Patients with T2–T3 distal rectal cancer had high-dose CRT to 60 Gy and additional endorectal brachytherapy boost of 5 Gy. Among 51 eligible patients, 40 had an initial clinical complete response and entered a watch and wait programme but of these 23% had local tumour regrowth. These results are in line with a report from Brazil including 81 patients with cT2N0 distal rectal cancer achieved cCR in 69% following CRT.[23] In the latter study period an extended CRT protocol including a 9 Gy boost and three cycles of consolidation chemotherapy after completion of RT a significantly higher cCR rate was obtained compared to standard CRT (85.7% vs. 56.6%, p <0.001).

Recently, the concept of total neoadjuvant therapy (TNT) was introduced.[24] This concept arises from the US, where many centres routinely prescribe postoperative chemotherapy following neoadjuvant CRT and surgery in rectal cancer. It has been observed that a significant proportion of patients do not receive the planned postoperative chemotherapy for various reasons (e.g. postoperative complications) and therefore one should aim to deliver all adjuvant therapy preoperatively. This concept is believed to increase the chances of organ preservation for rectal cancer patients. The OPRA trial demonstrated that CRT to a total of 50–56 Gy in combination with either induction or consolidation oxaliplatin/5-fluorouracil-based combination chemotherapy for four months yields organ preservation rates around 50% in stage II-III rectal cancer.[25]

Short-course radiotherapy

Hypofractionated short-course neoadjuvant RT for rectal cancer was largely pioneered in Sweden.[26] RT was administered in five fractions of five Gy in one week and surgery was scheduled the following week. With this regimen very little time was allowed for tumour response to RT and cCR rates could be expected to be very low. However, short-course radiotherapy (SCRT) has been shown to reduce local recurrence rates. In the Stockholm III trial one study arm consisted of SCRT with delayed surgery (4–6 weeks after completion of SCRT) and in that arm ypCR was observed in a significant proportion of patients (10.4%) indicating that also SCRT may be a valid option in in an organ preservation strategy.[4,6] These findings were substantiated by observational data from both Sweden and UK.

Having introduced a 'waiting period' between SCRT and surgery, a window of opportunity for also delivering chemotherapy preoperatively has emerged. This chemotherapy may be delivered at full-dose whereby an effect both on potentially present occult micrometastases and on the primary tumour could be expected. This approach was explored in a Polish trial reporting a ypCR rate of 16%.[12] In the Polish trial patients randomized to SCRT received three cycles of FOLFOX4 prior to surgery. In the RAPIDO trial in which 920 patients were randomized to either standard CRT or SCRT followed by six cycles of full-dose 5-FU and Oxaliplatin this concept is again tested.[27] Fewer treatment failures (23.7% vs. 30.4%) were seen in the experimental arm at 3 years, however, locoregional recurrence rates were higher in the experimental group (8.7% vs. 6%). Despite this, pathological complete response was higher in the experimental group (28% vs. 14%), with three-year overall survival similar between the groups (89% vs. 88.8%).[28]

External beam radiotherapy technique

Three-dimensional conformal radiotherapy uses CT scans for target delineation and dose planning. For improved precision, pelvic MRI can be merged with the dose-planning CT, and recently MRI for dose planning has become an alternative.

Guidelines have been developed for delineation of the clinical target volume (CTV) based on predominant location of local recurrences including different pelvic subsites and lymph node regions at risk of microscopic involvement.[29] The mesorectum, presacral space and lateral lymph nodes should always be included, and in case of T3 with extra-mesorectal nodes or T4 tumour also the external iliac nodes. The ischiorectal fossa should be included when the external sphincter or the ischiorectal fossa itself is involved, and should the sphincter apparatus or inferior third of the vagina be involved also the external inguinal nodes are to be included in the CTV.[30,31] The cranial and caudal CTV are defined according to tumour level and stage.

Until recently, conformal radiation technique with 3–4 fields has been commonly used, but increasingly more developed techniques such as intensity modulated radiotherapy (IMRT) and volumetric arc therapy (VMAT) are being utilized also for rectal cancer. The main advantages of the newer techniques are the precise dose delivery resulting in lower doses to the organs at risk (such as the small bowel), but also the possibility of simultaneous boost with higher doses to the gross tumour volume. Thus, less gastrointestinal and genitourinary toxicity and increased pCR rates can potentially be obtained. IMRT/VMAT is advantageous in locally advanced T4 rectal cancer with extended CTVs.

Brachytherapy

Endoluminal RT or brachytherapy is an option for treatment of rectal cancer, either alone or in combination with external beam radiotherapy (EBRT) and/or surgery.

Contact radiotherapy (Papillon technique) whereby very high doses can be delivered through a rectal applicator with a similar appearance to a rigid rectoscope is experiencing a renaissance following a new delivery system in 2008.[32] The technique is operator dependent and the delivery system is not universally available. In a significant proportion of patients with early tumours (T1) contact radiotherapy can achieve cCR but the technique may also be applicable for frail patients with more advanced lesions in whom surgery may not be an option. In combination with EBRT, cCR can also be obtained for T2–T3 tumours.[33] The OPERA trial in which contact radiotherapy was delivered either before or after CRT, depending on initial tumour size, reported cCR rates exceeding 80%.[34] With respect to assessment of response and follow-up experience is developing.[35]

An alternative brachytherapy technique is high-dose-rate endorectal brachytherapy (HDREBT) in which a flexible applicator is inserted transanally. Through eight peripheral channels HDR can be delivered with an ^{192}Ir source. In a Dutch phase I study designed to elucidate dose limiting toxicity, this technique was combined with EBRT in patients unfit for surgery, and 20 out of 33 patients experienced an initial cCR. With a median follow-up of 30 months 8 of 11 surviving patients were in complete remission.[36] A similar technique was used in a Danish study aiming to explore organ preservation for distal T2-T3N0-N1 tumours. Fifty-one patients were treated with CRT to 60 Gy followed by 5 Gy intracavitary brachytherapy, and 40 patients (78%) were classified as cCR. In addition, among seven patients who underwent surgery, two had ypCR.[22]

The techniques and experience reported in the literature suggest that there may be strategies where brachytherapy can serve as an adjunct to achieve cCR following CRT or SCRT in combination with chemotherapy. Increased rates of cCR may then be translated into improved organ preservation rates.

References

1. Glynne-Jones R, Wyrwicz L, Tiret E, et al. Rectal cancer: ESMO Clinical Practice Guidelines for diagnosis, treatment and follow-up. *Ann Oncol.* 2017: 1;28(suppl 4):iv22–iv40.
2. Glimelius B, Myklebust TÅ, Lundqvist K, et al. Two countries—two treatment strategies for rectal cancer. *Radiother Oncol.* 2016:121(3):357–63.
3. Morris EJ, Finan PJ, Spencer K, et al. Wide variation in the use of radiotherapy in the management of surgically treated rectal cancer across the English National Health Service. *Clin Oncol.* 2016: 28(8):522–31.

4. Erlandsson J, Holm T, Pettersson D, et al. Optimal fractionation of preoperative radiotherapy and timing to surgery for rectal cancer (Stockholm III): a multicentre, randomised, non-blinded, phase 3 non-inferiority trial. *Lancet Oncol.* 2017;18(3):336–46.
5. Braendengen M, Tveit KM, Berglund A, et al. Randomized phase III study comparing preoperative radiotherapy with chemotherapy in non-resectable rectal cancer. *J Clin Oncol.* 2008;26:3687–94.
6. Erlandsson J, Lörinc E, Ahlberg M, et al. Tumour regression after radiotherapy for rectal cancer—results from the randomized Stockholm III trial. *Radiother Oncol.* 2019;135:178–86.
7. Gerard JP, Azria D, Gourgou-Bourgade S, et al. Comparison of two neoadjubvant chemoradiotherapy regimens for locally advanced rectal cancer: results of the phase III trial ACCORD 12/0405-Prodige 2. *J Clin Oncol.* 2010;28:1638–44.
8. Aschele C, Cionini L, Lonardi S, et al. Primary tumour response to preoperative chemoradiation with or without oxaliplatin in locally advanced rectal cancer: Pathologic results of the STAR-01 randomized phase III trial. *J Clin Oncol.* 2011;29:2773–80.
9. Rödel C, Liersch T, Becker H, et al. Preoperative chemoradiotherapy and postoperative chemotherapy with fluorouracil and oxaliplatin versus fluorouracil alone in locally advanced rectal cancer: initial results of the German CAO/ARO/AIO-04 randomised phase-3 trial. *Lancet Oncol.* 2012;13:679–87.
10. Ngan SY, Burmeister B, Fisher RJ, et al. Randomized trial of short-course radiotherapy versus long-course chemoradiation comparing rates of local recurrence in patients with T3 rectal cancer: Trans-Tasmanian Radiation Oncology Group Trial 01.04. *J Clin Oncol.* 2012;30:3827–33.
11. O'Conell MJ, Colangelo LH, Beart RW, et al. Capecitabine and oxaliplatin in the preoperative multimodality treatment of rectal cancer: surgical end points from National Surgical Breast and Bowel Project trial R-04. *J Clin Oncol.* 2014;32:1927–34.
12. Bujko C, Wyrwicz L, Rutkowski A, et al. Long-course oxaliplatin-based preoperative chemoradiation versus 5x5 Gy and consolidation chemotherapy for cT4 or fixed cT3 rectal cancer: results of a randomized phase III study. *Ann Oncol.* 2016;27:834–42.
13. Lefevre JH, Mineur L, Kotti S, et al. Effect of interval (7 or 11 weeks) between neoadjuvant radiochemotherapy and surgery on complete pathologic response in rectal cancer: a multicenter, randomized controlled trial (GRECCAR-6). *J Clin Oncol.* 2016;34:3773–81.
14. Habr-Gama A, Perez RO, Nadalin W, et al. Operative versus non-operative treatment for stage 0 distal rectal cancer following chemoradiation therapy: long-term results. *Ann Surg.* 2014;240:711–17.
15. Dossa F, Chesney TR, Acuna SA, Baxter NN. A watch-and-wait approach for locally advanced rectal cancer after clinical complete response following neoadjuvant chemoradiation: a systemic review and meta-analysis. *Lancet Gastroenterol Hepatol.* 2017;2(7):501–13.
16. van der Valk MJM, Hilling DE, Bastiaannet E, et al. Long-term outcomes of clinical complete responders after neoadjuvant treatment for rectal cancer in the International Watch & Wait Database (IWWD): an international multicentre registry study. *Lancet.* 2018;391:2537–45.
17. Sauer R, Becker H, Hohenberger W, et al. Preoperative versus postoperative chemoradiotherapy for rectal cancer. *N Engl J Med.* 2004;351:1731–40.
18. Bosset JF, Collette L, Calais G, et al. Chemotherapy with preoperative radiotherapy in rectal cancer. *N Engl J Med.* 2006;355:1114–23.
19. Guren MG, Kørner H, Pfeffer F, et al. Nationwide improvement of rectal cancer treatment outcomes in Norway, 1993–2010. *Acta Oncol.* 2015;54:1714–22.

20. Dewdney A, Cunningham D, Tabernero J, et al. Multicenter randomized phase II clinical trial comparing neoadjuvant oxaliplatin, capicetabine and preoperative radiotherapy with or without cetuximab followed by total mesorectal excision in high-risk rectal cancer (EXPERT-C). *J Clin Oncol.* 2012;30(14):1620–27.
21. Chua YJ, Barbachano Y, Cunningham D, et al. Neoadjuvant capecitabine and oxaliplatin before chemoradiotherapy and total mesorectaöl excision in MRI-defined poor-risk rectal cancer: a phase II trial. *Lancet Oncol.* 2010;11(3):241–8.
22. Appelt A, Pløen J, Harling H, et al. High-dose chemoradiotherapy and watchful waiting for distal rectal cancer: a prospective observational study. *Lancet Oncol.* 2015;16(8):919–27.
23. Habr-Gama A, São Julião GP, Vailati BB, et al. Organ preservation in cT2N0 rectal cancer after neoadjuvant chemoradiation therapy: the impact of radiation therapy dose-escalation and consolidation chemotherapy. *Ann Surg.* 2019;269:102–7.
24. Ludmir EB, Palta M, Willett CG, et al. Total neoadjuvant therapy for rectal cancer: an emerging option. *Cancer.* 2017;123(9):1497–506.
25. Garcia-Aguilar J, Patil S, Gollub MJ, et al. Organ preservation in patients with rectal adenocarcinoma treated with total neoadjuvant therapy. *J Clin Oncol.* 2022;40:2546–57.
26. Anonymous. Improved survival with preoperative radiotherapy in resectable rectal cancer: Swedish Rectal Cancer Trial. *N Engl J Med.* 1997;336(14):980–7.
27. Nilsson PJ, et al. Short-course radiotherapy followed by neo-adjuvant chemotherapy in locally advanced rectal cancer—the RAPIDO trial. *BMC Cancer.* 2013;13:279.
28. Bahadoer R, Dijkstra EA, van Etten B, et al. Short-course radiotherapy followed by chemotherapy before total mesorectal excision (TME) versus preoperative chemoradiotherapy, TME and optional adjuvant chemotherapy in locally advanced rectal cancer (RAPIDO): a randomised, open-label, phase 3 trial. *Lancet Oncol.* 2021;22(1):29–42.
29. Roels S, Duthoy W, Haustermans K, et al. Definition and delineation of the clinical target volume for rectal cancer. *Int J Radiat Oncol Biol Phys.* 2006;65:1129–42.
30. Myerson RJ, Garofalo MC, El Naqa I, et al. Elective clinical target volumes for conformal therapy in anorectal cancer: a radiation therapy oncology group consensus panel contouring atlas. *Int J Radiat Oncol Biol Phys.* 2009;74:824–30.
31. Valentino V, Gambacorta MA, Barbaro B, et al. International consensus guidelines on Clinical Target Volume delineation in rectal cancer. *Radiother Oncol.* 2016;120(2):195–201.
32. Gerard JP, Myint AS, Croce O, et al. Renaissance of contact x-ray therapy for treating rectal cancer. *Exp Rev Med Devices.* 2011;8:483–92.
33. Frin AC, Evesque L, Gal J, et al. Organ or sphincter preservation for rectal cancer. The role of contact x-ray brachytherapy in a monocentric series of 112 patients. *Eur J Cancer.* 2017;72:124–36.
34. Gerard JP, Barbet N, Schiappa R, et al. Neoadjuvant chemoradiotherapy with radiation dose escalation with contact x-ray brachytherapy boost or external beam radiotherapy boost for organ preservation in early cT2-cT3 rectal adenocarcinoma (OPERA): a phase 3, randomised controlled trial. *Lancet Gastroenterol Hepatol.* 2023;4:356–67.
35. Dunstan MJD, Rockall TA, Potter K, Stewart AJ. Radiological and clinical findings following rectal contact x-ray brachytherapy (Papillon technique)—how to assess response. *J Contemp Brachyther.* 2018;10:179–89.
36. Rijkmans EC, Cats A, Nout RA, et al. Endo rectal brachytherapy boost after external beam radiation therapy in elderly or medically inoperable patients with rectal cancer: primary outcomes of the phase 1 HERBERT Study. *Int J Radiat Oncol Biol Phys.* 2017;98:908–17.

4

Time interval to surgery and its impact on complete response rates in locally advanced rectal cancer

Maxime K. Collard and Jérémie H. Lefèvre

Rectal cancer is among the commonest cancers worldwide.[1] When diagnosed at a non-metastatic stage of disease, more than half of patients have locally advanced rectal cancer, including invasion of the mesorectum by the tumour and/or metastatic lymph nodes.[2] In the early 1990s, several randomized trials demonstrated the benefit of a combining chemotherapy, radiotherapy and a surgical approach for T3/T4 or N+ rectal cancers.[3,4] While preoperative RCT has become the standard treatment for stage II and III rectal cancer,[5,6] the optimal delay between the end of radiotherapy (RT) and surgery is still debated. This delay strongly influences the percentage of pathological complete response (pCR).[7] pCR represents the perfect outcome of neoadjuvant therapy, with it being associated with improved survival and decreased local recurrence.[8–10] The aim of this chapter is to present and analyse the complex and sometimes contradictory data in the literature concerning the optimum delay after RT or RCT.

Time interval to surgery and cellular biology

It is essential to understand the different mechanisms of RT on rectal cancer at the cellular level to establish whether there is radiobiological evidence that increasing the delay after RT can increase tumour cell mortality.

Although some cells in recently irradiated tumour tissue have a morphologically normal appearance, these cells are destined to die due to the damage caused by ionizing radiation.[11] At the cellular level, the effectiveness of RT is based on several mechanisms. Firstly, radiation-induced DNA damage is the direct toxicity of ionizing radiation on the DNA of tumour cells, inducing their mortality. This pathway is direct and cell death is rapid.[12] Secondly, cell mortality is also induced by indirect mechanisms of action, which can potentially be delayed such as locally released reactive oxygen species (ROS) following irradiation which play a role in tumour cell death. These ROS can persist at the operative site and induce senescence and delayed cell death over time.[13] Other mechanisms of delayed action are also involved, such as changes in peritumoural immunity, which is a sequential process that evolves over time.[14]

In addition to the complexity of the different anti-tumour mechanisms induced by RT on the irradiated zone, there is also an 'abscopal effect', which is an anti-tumour effect at a distance from the irradiated tumour. In fact, irradiated tumour cells induce activation of the immune system, predominantly via antigen-presenting cells. This activation of the immune system at the irradiation site triggers an anti-tumour immune reaction away from the irradiated lesion.[15] The abscopal effect of RT is not immediate, and may justify prolonging the interval between RT and surgery in patients with rectal cancer. Although the abscopal effect of RT in rectal cancer theoretically exists, it has never been demonstrated in practice for this cancer.[16]

Although increasing the delay between RT and surgery may have benefits for the indirect cell death mechanisms, it can be dangerous for two reasons. Firstly, there is a risk of tumour regrowth if some tumour cells are resistant to RT. Secondarily, lengthening the delay between RT and surgery increases the delay between RT and postoperative adjuvant chemotherapy, potentially leaving micrometastasis untreated, leading to increased rates of metastatic disease Finally, lengthening the delay may increase the fibrosis in the pelvis leading to difficulty pelvic dissection.

Radiochemotherapy and delayed proctectomy: historic studies

The Lyon R90-01 randomized controlled trial was the first prospective randomized trial to evaluate the value of extending the delay between neoadjuvant RT (39 Gy in 13 fractions) and surgery in rectal cancer.[17] When surgery was performed 6 to 8 weeks after RT (long interval), the histological response (pCR or few residual tumour cells) was significantly increased compared to the group that underwent surgery 2 weeks after RT (26% and 10%, respectively, $p = 0.005$). However, the long interval did not provide any benefit in regard to morbidity, local relapse, sphincter-preserving surgery, or short-term survival between the two groups. Publication of the long-term results of this trial after 17 years of follow-up did not show any differences in the local recurrence rate or overall survival between the long-interval group and the short-interval group.[18] Despite the lack of survival benefit, this study demonstrated for the first time the benefit of extending the time between RT and surgery in patients with rectal cancer, specifically an improved histological response. This delay of 6–7 weeks became the standard of care.

After the publication of this prospective randomized trial, several new approaches were developed, including the concomitant addition of fluoropyrimidine-based chemotherapy (5FU or capecitabine) to RT according to the long-term 45–50 Gy protocol. In particular, the addition of this concomitant chemotherapy was found to significantly increase the rate of pCR compared to RT alone when using the long protocol (45–50 Gy).[19] The application of combined neoadjuvant RT treatment and fluoropyrimidine chemotherapy followed by proctectomy 6 to 8 weeks later has become the gold standard treatment for T3, T4, and N+ rectal cancer. Notably, this delay of 6 to 8 weeks between neoadjuvant treatment (RT and chemotherapy) and surgery has not been validated by a prospective randomized phase III comparative trial.

Many consecutive retrospective studies have aimed to answer the question: can we increase the rate of pCR by increasing the time between RCT and surgery? Probst et al. retrospectively analysed the American National Cancer Data Base involving 17,255 patients with a clinical stage II and III rectal cancer treated by RCT and then surgery.[20] This study showed a significant increase in the pCR rate with time (<6 weeks 8.7% vs. >8 weeks 13.2% (p <0.001). However, the interval between 6 and 8 weeks after the RCT is the decisive period, considering the pCR rate was already 11.7%. Probst and Kalady published in their respective study the same sigmoid curves showing that the major effect of radiotherapy occurs around 6–8 weeks (Fig. 4.1).[7,20]

In order to synthesize the findings of the numerous retrospective studies about the best delay between RCT and surgery, a meta-analysis of 19,652 patients found that an increased delay between neoadjuvant treatment and surgery of more than 8 weeks conferred a significant improvement on the rate of patients with pCR (risk ratio = 1.25, [1.16–1.35]; p <0.0001).[22] This meta-analysis classified patients into only two groups based on the time interval between RCT and surgery: less than 8 weeks versus more than 8 weeks. Among patients with a delay greater than 8 weeks, some waited 9 weeks while others waited until 14 weeks, for instance, which introduces a source of heterogeneity within the same group that should not be overlooked. Similarly, among the patients with a delay of less than 8 weeks some waited only 4 weeks while others waited 7 weeks. As exposed previously in Figure 4.1, the crucial delay seems to be between 6 and 8 weeks, so that the heterogeneity within the group with a delay of less than 8 weeks is problematic. To clarify this point, a further meta-analysis analysed the difference between delays of 5 and 12 weeks.[23] Although the number of studies evaluating each of the thresholds was not similar, this meta-analysis concluded that the best interval to optimize the rate of pCR is 7 or 8 weeks (risk ratio = 1.45; risk ratio of 1.49). In this work, patients with a delay of 10 or 12 weeks showed no increase in the rate of pCR.

Although the synthesis of these meta-analyses is relatively difficult, despite the large number of patients analysed. The main message is that the short delay <6 weeks seems deleterious on the rate of pCR while the majority of the patients achieve a pCR between 7–8 weeks.

Prospective, randomized studies

The GRECCAR6 prospective, multicentre, randomized controlled trial conducted in France is the first trial to evaluate the benefit of extending the post-RCT period to more than 6–8 weeks.[25] In this study, 265 patients with cT3/T4 or TxN+ cancers of the lower or middle rectum were randomized to a 7- or 11-week interval after standardized RCT (45–50 Gy + fluorouracil or capecitabine). The proportion of patients in pCR, was similar between the two groups (15.0% and 17.4% for 7 and 11 weeks, respectively, p = 0.5983). In addition, patients in the 11-week group experienced

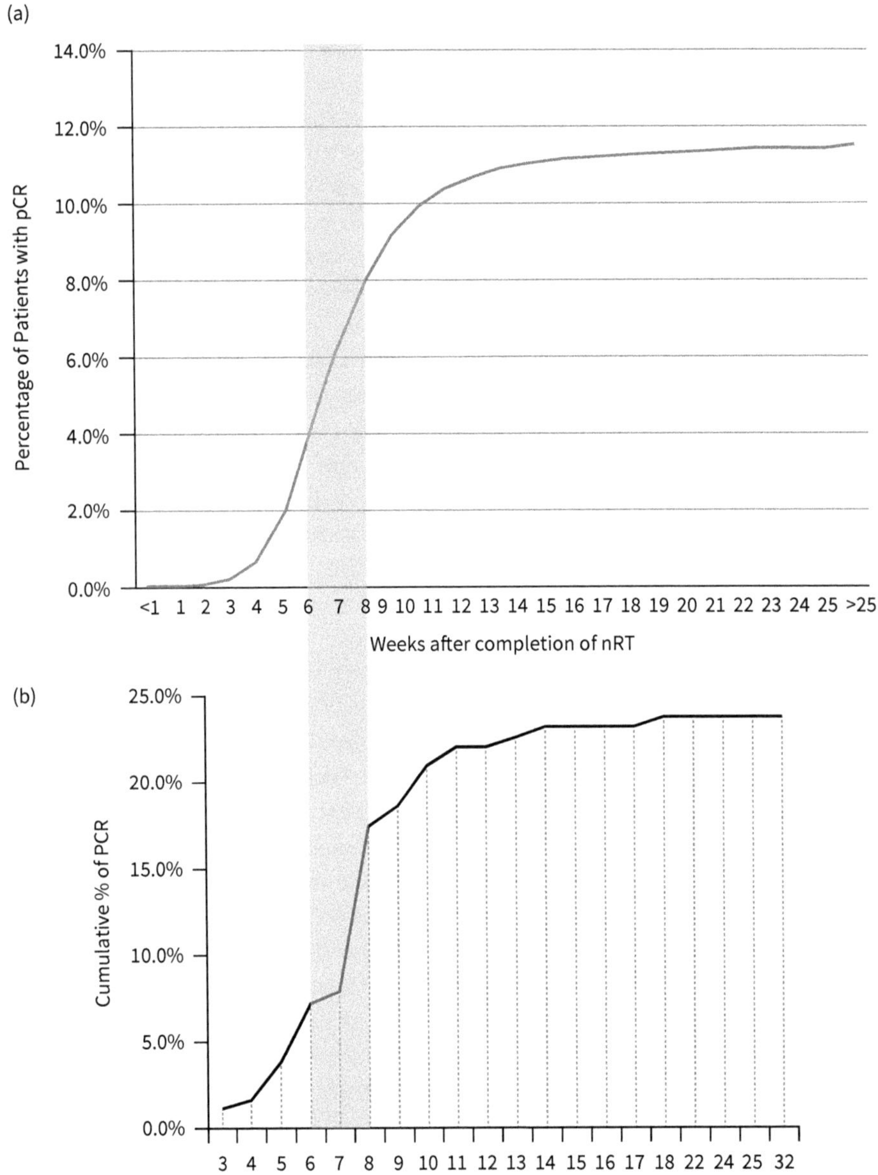

Fig. 4.1 Evolution of the rate of pCR according to the interval between the RCT and the surgery: the crucial period of 6–8 weeks.
Sourced from 1A: Probst et al. *J Am Coll Surg*. (2015)[20]; 1B: Kalady et al. *Ann Surg*. (2009).[7]

significant increases in postoperative morbidity (45% vs. 32%, $p = 0.0404$) due to medical complications (32.8% vs. 19.2%, $p = 0.0137$), and worse mesorectal resection quality (21% vs. 10%, $p = 0.0156$). Thus, the overall results of this work do not support an increase in the delay to 11 weeks. Interestingly, the metastatic progression of the disease during the waiting period was a rare event and did not rise when the waiting time was increased (2.3% in the 7-week group and 1.5% in the 11-week group).

In parallel with this French trial, a prospective randomized controlled trial conducted by the Royal Marsden Hospital team in London compared the downstaging, pCR and TRG1-2 rates between patients who waited 6 versus 12 weeks between the end of RCT and surgery.[26] The results from this trial are the opposite of those from the GRECCAR6 trial, where the proportion of pathological downstaging was significantly increased in the 12-week group (58%) compared to the 6-week group (43%, $p = 0.019$). The pCR rate was lower in the 6-week group versus the 12-week group (9% and 20%, respectively, $p < 0.05$). Of course, it is surprising that these two well-conducted phase III trials with a high level of evidence found opposite results. However, it is important to note that the primary endpoint of the British trial was the downstaging evaluated by MRI (mrTRG). Thus, the pCR was a secondary endpoint, with the resulting biases due to the fact that sample size calculation was not based on this pathological criterion. In the British trial, the pCR rate in the 6-week group was only 9% while it was 20% at 12 weeks. In the GRECCAR 6 trial, the rate of pCR was already 15% for the 7 weeks group and did not increase for the 11-week group. Thus, as suggested by retrospective studies and meta-analyses, it is between 6 and 8 weeks that the pCR is obtained, and this percentage remains stable beyond this time.

A third prospective randomized controlled trial on the subject has been conducted by a Turkish team,[27] which can be differentiated from the other two prospective randomized trials by at least two points. Firstly, this trial was conducted at a single centre, and all patients were operated by the same two surgeons. Secondly, the definition of the short interval and the long interval between RCT and surgery was not defined by a specific timepoint but by a period, where randomized patients in the short-interval group had a delay of between 4 and 8 weeks while the long-interval group had a delay of between 8 and 12 weeks. A total of 160 patients were randomized in the short-interval group and 167 in the long-interval group, with a mean delay between the end of RCT and the surgery of 46.1 ± 7.3 days for the short-interval group and 71.1 ± 9.3 days for the long-interval group. The pCR rate was significantly higher in the long-interval group compared to the short-interval group (10.0% vs. 18.6%, $p = 0.027$). It is important to note that a multivariate analysis of the factors associated with pCR did not find the long interval to be statistically associated with pCR. The choice of a delay between 4 and 8 weeks for the short-term group makes it difficult to interpret the results of this trial. Indeed, retrospective and prospective studies suggest that it is between the sixth and eighth weeks that the pCR occurs. Thus, having in the same group patients operated after a period of four weeks and after a period of seven weeks constitutes a limit of this trial. In our opinion, the heterogeneity of the groups concerning the delay between the RCT and the surgery does not lead to the conclusion that extending the delay to more than 8 weeks improves the pCR rate.

GRECCAR6 trial has since published three-year oncological outcomes. Interestingly, randomization had no influence on three-year OS ($p = 0.8868$) or disease-free survival (DFS) ($p = 0.9409$). Distant ($p = 0.7432$) and local ($p = 0.3944$) recurrences were also not influenced by increasing the interval to surgery. DFS was independently influenced by three factors: circumferential radial margin (CRM) ≤1 mm

(HR= 2.03), ypT3-T4 (HR = 2.69), and positive lymph nodes (HR = 3.62). Thus, increasing the interval by four weeks had no influence on oncological outcomes.[29]

Increasing pCR with smaller tumour and delayed surgery?

In the era of rectal preservation, several studies have evaluated the efficacy of RCT on earlier stage tumours. Garcia-Aguilar et al. obtained a ypT0 rate of 44% in cT2N0 patients with a surgery performed only six weeks after the RCT.[30] Similarly, the GRECCAR2 study, including patients with small rectal cancers (cT2/T3 of maximum size 4 cm) found five weeks after the RCT a ypT0 rate of 40%. This suggests that the size of the irradiated tumour is a major factor in obtaining a pCR more than the lengthening of the delay between cardiac resynchronization therapy (CRT) and surgery. In these cases, 6–7 weeks seems enough to reach a high pCR rate.

Interval between a short radiotherapy protocol and proctectomy

While the optimum delay after a long RCT protocol (45–50 Gy + fluorouracil or capecitabine) to obtain the best rate of pCR in patients has been the subject of many studies, this problem has not been overly considered for the short 25 Gy RT protocol (5×5 Gy over 1 week) as the objective of this protocol is not to achieve downstaging.[31] However, some prospective trials have shown that this 25 Gy RT protocol is able to induce tumour regression despite the short delay of only 1 week.[32,33] In addition, some retrospective studies have highlighted the potential value of prolonging the delay after RT with 25 Gy in order to improve the outcomes, particularly the histological results.[34,35] Veenhof et al. published a prospective, non-randomized study comparing a short delay of 1 week to a long delay of 6–8 weeks after 25 Gy RT (5×5 Gy over 1 week).[36] Prolonging the delay in this context was associated with significant increases in the pCR rate (12% vs. 0%) and the downstaging rate (55% vs. 26%).

Following this work, two prospective randomized trials have been published.[37,38] In the study conducted by Pach et al., 77 patients were randomized into the short-interval group (5–7 days) and 77 patients into the long-interval group (4–5 weeks).[37] This trial, which presented a high level of evidence, showed a significant benefit on downstaging in the long-interval group (44% vs. 13%, $p = 0.0001$), as well as an improved pCR rate (10.4% vs. 0%, $p = 0.003$). The second published trial was the interim analysis of the Stockholm III trial, which compared a short-interval group (1 week) with a long-interval group (4–8 weeks).[38] The results of this study were in agreement with the other trials on this subject, showing a significant benefit on the rate of pCR in favour of the long-interval group (11.8%) compared to the short-interval group (1.7%; $p = 0.001$). The final survival outcomes of this phase III non-inferiority trial were recently published, demonstrating non-inferiority of the long interval versus the short interval regarding overall survival, local recurrence, and recurrent disease.[39] In addition, the rates of postoperative complications and surgical complications were significantly reduced in the long-interval group.

As summarized in Table 4.2 (see also Table 4.1), all prospective studies agree on the benefit of lengthening the delay after the 5 × 5 Gy RT protocol from 1 week to more

Table 4.1 Systematic review of prospective randomized controlled trials assessing the benefit of increasing the interval between radiochemotherapy (45–50 Gy + fluorouracil or capecitabine) and surgery on the pCR

	Year	Number of patients	Interval between RCT and surgery	pCR[3]	Complete resection of the mesorectum	Postoperative morbidity
Lefèvre et al.[25]	2016	n = 265 SI[1:] n = 133 LI[2:] n = 132	SI: 7 weeks LI: 11 weeks	SI: 15.0% LI: 17.4% $p = 0.598$	SI: 84.3% LI: 90.0% $p = 0.016$	SI: 32.0% LI: 44.5% $p = 0.04$
Evans et al.[26]	2016	n = 237 SI: n = 122 LI: n = 115	SI: 6 weeks LI: 12 weeks	SI: 9% LI: 20% $p < 0.05$	*	*
Akgun et al.[27]	2018	n = 327 SI: n = 160 LI: n = 167	SI: 4–8 weeks LI: 8–12 weeks	SI: 10.0% LI: 18.6% $p = 0.027$	SI: 90.0% LI: 89.2% $p = 0.713$	SI: 22.5% LI: 19.8% $p = 0.305$

[1]SI, short interval; [2]LI, long interval; [3]pCR, pathological complete response; *study not yet published, data not available.

Table 4.2 Systematic review of prospective controlled trials assessing the benefit of increasing the interval between radiotherapy alone 25 Gy (5 × 5 Gy over a week) and surgery on the pCR

	Year	Randomization	Number of patients	Interval between RCT and surgery	pCR[3]	5-year overall survival
Veenhof et al.[36]	2006	No	n = 108 SI[1:] n = 57 LI[2:] n = 151	SI: 2 weeks LI: 6–8 weeks	SI: 0% LI: 12% $\mathbf{p < 0.01}$	SI: 66.4% LI: 73.3% $p = 0.12$
Pach et al.[37]	2012	Yes	n = 154 SI: n = 77 LI: n = 77	SI: 7–10 days LI: 4–5 weeks	SI: 0% LI: 10.4% $\mathbf{p = 0.003}$	SI: 63% LI: 73% $p = 0.24$
Pettersson et al.[38]	2015	Yes	n = 462 SI: n = 234 LI: n = 228	SI: 4–8 weeks LI: 8–12 weeks	SI: 11.8% LI: 1.7% $\mathbf{p = 0.001}$	–

[1]SI, short interval; [2]LI, long interval; [3]pCR, pathological complete response.

than 4 weeks on the rate of pCR in patients with rectal cancer, although a benefit on the local recurrence rate or survival could not be demonstrated.

Increasing the delay between radiochemotherapy and surgery: an opportunity for consolidation neoadjuvant chemotherapy?

It has been shown previously that increasing the delay between cancer diagnosis and surgery is an independent factor that alters overall survival.[40] The problem with lengthening the period between RCT and surgery is therefore linked to tumour proliferation, which is not controlled by initial RCT. However, administering chemotherapy in the waiting period between the end of RCT and surgery. allows a long delay between RCT and surgery, thereby maximizing the efficiency of ionizing radiation while also controlling tumour proliferation during this period. [41] With this strategy, the proportion of patients in pCR could be improved.

A multicentre, non-randomized phase II study evaluated the efficacy of FOLFOX chemotherapy on patients' histological response in the interval between RCT and surgery.[42] All patients received neoadjuvant RCT, with four groups being evaluated: group 1 were operated 6 weeks after RCT, group 2 were operated 12 weeks after RCT and received two cycles of FOLFOX during this interval, group 3 were operated 16 weeks after RCT and received four cycles of FOLFOX during this interval, and group 4 were operated 20 weeks after RCT and received six cycles of FOLFOX during this interval. The rate of pCR increased with the number of cycles of FOLFOX, with 18% in group 1, 25% in group 2, 30% in group 3, and 38% in group 4 ($p = 0.0036$). As expected, the proportion of patients who experienced adverse events during FOLFOX treatment increased from group 2 to group 4. The results of this phase II trial highlights the benefit of combined chemotherapy when extending the time between CRT and surgery on the pCR response rate, but this significantly increased chemotherapy-related toxicity. The WAIT randomized controlled trial compared the pCR between a 10-week group of patients treated with RCT and a 10-week group of patients treated with RCT who received three cycles of 5-fluorouracil and leucovorin during this waiting period. [43] The results of this trial were unremarkable, with a similar rate of patients in pCR between the two groups ($p = 0.49$). It is clear that the effectiveness of interval chemotherapy for potentiating the benefit of a long delay between neoadjuvant RCT and surgery depends on the type of chemotherapy and the number of cycles. A Korean phase III trial on this topic is currently in progress, evaluating a more aggressive chemotherapy regimen including three cycles of FOLFOX.[44] This trial uses a similar duration between neoadjuvant RCT and nine-week surgery, so the results of this work will likely provide some answers about the suspected benefit of chemotherapy between RCT and surgery.

Conclusion

In conclusion, this work synthesizes the complex data regarding the optimum delay between neoadjuvant RCT or RT alone and surgery. A number of factors must be considered, such as the total dose of RT, its fractionation, the tumour size, and the possible association with

Chemotherapy during the waiting period. Regarding the short 25 Gy RT protocol, it seems that the traditional one-week delay can be extended to four weeks to ensure a better rate of pCR, although there is no evidence of improved patient survival. After a conventional long-term protocol (45–50 Gy + fluorouracil or capecitabine) the best pCR rate is obtained seven to eight weeks after the RCT. The interval must not be lengthened to excess in an attempt to improve the effectiveness of RT, as the progression of tumour cells surpasses the effect of RT after a certain delay. It is possible that the addition of chemotherapy during this interval in the future may play an important role in controlling the risk of tumour proliferation in the waiting period between neoadjuvant RCT and surgery. The future rests upon the mutational profile of the tumour, which will allow the selection of a delay according to the probability of response of the tumour.[45]

References

1. Torre LA, Bray F, Siegel RL, et al. Global cancer statistics, 2012. *CA Cancer J Clin.* 2015;65:87–108.
2. Kozak KR, Moody JS. The impact of T and N stage on long-term survival of rectal cancer patients in the community. *J Surg Oncol.* 2008;98:161–6.
3. Douglass HO, Moertel CG, Mayer RJ, et al. Survival after postoperative combination treatment of rectal cancer. *N Engl J Med.* 1986;315:1294–5.
4. Krook JE, Moertel CG, Gunderson LL, et al. Effective surgical adjuvant therapy for high-risk rectal carcinoma. *N Engl J Med.* 1991;324:709–15.
5. Lakkis Z, Manceau G, Bridoux V, et al. Management of rectal cancer: the 2016 French guidelines. *Colorectal Dis.* 2017;19:115–22.
6. Glynne-Jones R, Wyrwicz L, Tiret E, et al. Rectal cancer: ESMO Clinical Practice guidelines for diagnosis, treatment and follow-up. *Ann Oncol.* 2017;28:iv22–iv40.
7. Kalady MF, de Campos-Lobato LF, Stocchi L, et al. Predictive factors of pathologic complete response after neoadjuvant chemoradiation for rectal cancer. *Ann Surg.* 2009;250:582–9.
8. Theodoropoulos G, Wise WE, Padmanabhan A, et al. T-level downstaging and complete pathologic response after preoperative chemoradiation for advanced rectal cancer result in decreased recurrence and improved disease-free survival. *Dis Colon Rectum.* 2002;45:895–903.
9. Rödel C, Martus P, Papadoupolos T, et al. Prognostic significance of tumor regression after preoperative chemoradiotherapy for rectal cancer. *J Clin Oncol.* 2005;23:8688–96.
10. Kuo L-J, Liu M-C, Jian JJ-M, et al. Is final TNM staging a predictor for survival in locally advanced rectal cancer after preoperative chemoradiation therapy? *Ann Surg Oncol.* 2007;14:2766–72.

11. Suit HD, Gallager HS. Intact tumor cells in irradiated tissue. *Arch Pathol.* 1964;78:648–51.
12. Lomax ME, Folkes LK, O'Neill P. Biological consequences of radiation-induced DNA damage: relevance to radiotherapy. *Clin Oncol.* 2013;25:578–85.
13. Schaue D, McBride WH. Opportunities and challenges of radiotherapy for treating cancer. *Nat Rev Clin Oncol.* 2015;12:527–40.
14. Schaue D, McBride WH. Links between innate immunity and normal tissue radiobiology. *Radiat Res.* 2010;173:406–17.
15. Grass GD, Krishna N, Kim S. The immune mechanisms of abscopal effect in radiation therapy. *Curr Probl Cancer.* 2016;40:10–24.
16. Abuodeh Y, Venkat P, Kim S. Systematic review of case reports on the abscopal effect. *Curr Probl Cancer.* 2016;40:25–37.
17. Francois Y, Nemoz CJ, Baulieux J, et al. Influence of the interval between preoperative radiation therapy and surgery on downstaging and on the rate of sphincter-sparing surgery for rectal cancer: the Lyon R90-01 randomized trial. *J Clin Oncol.* 1999;17:2396.
18. Glehen O, Chapet O, Adham M, et al. Long-term results of the Lyons R randomized trial of preoperative radiotherapy with delayed surgery and its effect on sphincter-saving surgery in rectal cancer. *Br J Surg.* 2003;90:996–8.
19. Gérard J-P, Conroy T, Bonnetain F, et al. Preoperative radiotherapy with or without concurrent fluorouracil and leucovorin in T3–4 rectal cancers: results of FFCD 9203. *J Clin Oncol.* 2006;24:4620–5.
20. Probst CP, Becerra AZ, Aquina CT, et al. Extended intervals after neoadjuvant therapy in locally advanced rectal cancer: the key to improved tumor response and potential organ preservation. *J Am Coll Surg.* 2015;221:430–40.
21. Petrelli F, Sgroi G, Sarti E, et al. Increasing the interval between neoadjuvant chemoradiotherapy and surgery in rectal cancer: a meta-analysis of published studies. *Ann Surg.* 2016;263:458–64.
22. Du D, Su Z, Wang D, et al. Optimal interval to surgery after neoadjuvant chemoradiotherapy in rectal cancer: a systematic review and meta-analysis. *Clin Colorectal Cancer.* 2018;17:13–24.
23. Wang X-J, Zheng Z-R, Chi P, et al. Effect of interval between neoadjuvant chemoradiotherapy and surgery on oncological outcome for rectal cancer: a systematic review and meta-analysis. *Gastroenterol Res Pract.* 2016;2016:6756859.
24. Yang Y-J, Cao L, Li Z-W, et al. Fluorouracil-based neoadjuvant chemoradiotherapy with or without oxaliplatin for treatment of locally advanced rectal cancer: an updated systematic review and meta-analysis. *Oncotarget.* 2016;7:45513–24.
25. Lefevre JH, Mineur L, Kotti S, et al. Effect of interval (7 or 11 weeks) between neoadjuvant radiochemotherapy and surgery on complete pathologic response in rectal cancer: a multicenter, randomized, controlled trial (GRECCAR-6). *J Clin Oncol.* 2016;34:3773–80.
26. Evans J, Bhoday J, Sizer B, et al. Results of a prospective randomised control 6 vs 12 trial: is greater tumour downstaging observed on post treatment MRI if surgery is delayed to 12-weeks versus 6-weeks after completion of neoadjuvant chemoradiotherapy? *Ann Oncol.* 2016;27(suppl 6).
27. Akgun E, Caliskan C, Bozbiyik O, et al. Randomized clinical trial of short or long interval between neoadjuvant chemoradiotherapy and surgery for rectal cancer. *Br J Surg.* 2018;105:1417–25.
28. Denost Q, Rouanet P, Faucheron J-L, et al. To drain or not to drain infraperitoneal anastomosis after rectal excision for cancer: the GRECCAR 5 randomized trial. *Ann Surg.* 2017;265:474–80.
29. Lefèvre JH, Mineur L, Cachanado M, et al. Does a longer waiting period after neoadjuvant radio-chemotherapy improve the oncological prognosis of rectal cancer? Three

years' follow-up results of the GRECCAR-6 randomized multicenter trial. *Ann Surg.* 2019;270:747–54.

30. Garcia-Aguilar J, Shi Q, Thomas CR, et al. A phase II trial of neoadjuvant chemoradiation and local excision for T2N0 rectal cancer: preliminary results of the ACOSOG Z6041 trial. *Ann Surg Oncol.* 2012;19:384–91.
31. Marijnen CA, Nagtegaal ID, Klein Kranenbarg E, et al. No downstaging after short-term preoperative radiotherapy in rectal cancer patients. *J Clin Oncol.* 2001;19:1976–84.
32. Swedish Rectal Cancer Trial, Cedermark B, Dahlberg M, et al. Improved survival with preoperative radiotherapy in resectable rectal cancer. *N Engl J Med.* 1997;336:980–7.
33. Sebag-Montefiore D, Stephens RJ, Steele R, et al. Preoperative radiotherapy versus selective postoperative chemoradiotherapy in patients with rectal cancer (MRC CR07 and NCIC-CTG C016): a multicentre, randomised trial. *Lancet.* 2009;373:811–20.
34. Radu C, Berglund A, Påhlman L, et al. Short-course preoperative radiotherapy with delayed surgery in rectal cancer—a retrospective study. *Radiother Oncol.* 2008;87:343–9.
35. Pettersson D, Holm T, Iversen H, et al. Preoperative short-course radiotherapy with delayed surgery in primary rectal cancer. *Br J Surg.* 2012;99:577–83.
36. Veenhof AAFA, Kropman RHJ, Engel AF, et al. Preoperative radiation therapy for locally advanced rectal cancer: a comparison between two different time intervals to surgery. *Int J Colorectal Dis.* 2007;22:507–13.
37. Pach R, Kulig J, Richter P, et al. Randomized clinical trial on preoperative radiotherapy 25 Gy in rectal cancer—treatment results at 5-year follow-up. *Langenbecks Arch Surg.* 2012;397:801–7.
38. Pettersson D, Lörinc E, Holm T, et al. Tumour regression in the randomized Stockholm III Trial of radiotherapy regimens for rectal cancer. *Br J Surg.* 2015;102:972–8.
39. Erlandsson J, Holm T, Pettersson D, et al. Optimal fractionation of preoperative radiotherapy and timing to surgery for rectal cancer (Stockholm III): a multicentre, randomised, non-blinded, phase 3, non-inferiority trial. *Lancet Oncol.* 2017;18:336–46.
40. Supiot S, Bennouna J, Rio E, et al. Negative influence of delayed surgery on survival after preoperative radiotherapy in rectal cancer. *Colorectal Dis.* 2006;8:430–5.
41. Habr-Gama A, Perez RO, Sabbaga J, et al. Increasing the rates of complete response to neoadjuvant chemoradiotherapy for distal rectal cancer: results of a prospective study using additional chemotherapy during the resting period. *Dis Colon Rectum.* 2009;52:1927–34.
42. Garcia-Aguilar J, Chow OS, Smith DD, et al. Effect of adding mFOLFOX6 after neoadjuvant chemoradiation in locally advanced rectal cancer: a multicentre, phase 2 trial. *Lancet Oncol.* 2015;16:957–66.
43. Moore J, Price T, Carruthers S, et al. Prospective randomized trial of neoadjuvant chemotherapy during the 'wait period' following preoperative chemoradiotherapy for rectal cancer: results of the WAIT trial. *Colorectal Dis.* 2017;19:973–9.
44. Kim CW, Kang BM, Kim IY, et al. Korean Society of Coloproctology (KSCP) trial of cONsolidation Chemotherapy for Locally advanced mid or low rectal cancer after neoadjUvant concurrent chemoraDiothErapy: a multicenter, randomized controlled trial (KONCLUDE). *BMC Cancer.* 2018;18:538.
45. Bengala C, Bettelli S, Bertolini F, et al. Prognostic role of EGFR gene copy number and KRAS mutation in patients with locally advanced rectal cancer treated with preoperative chemoradiotherapy. *Br J Cancer.* 2010;103:1019–24.

5

Total neoadjuvant therapy in locally advanced rectal cancer

Eva L.K. Voogt, Harm J.T. Rutten, Miranda Kusters, and Pim J.W.A. Burger

Introduction

Over the past decades, there have been significant developments in the treatment of rectal cancer however, the introduction of total mesorectal excision (TME) by Heald et al.[1] refined surgical technique and led to a decrease in both involved surgical margins as well as local recurrence rates.[2] To further improve these results, the administration of radiotherapy as a complementary treatment to the surgical treatment of locally advanced rectal cancer (LARC) also evolved during the years. In the pre-TME era, chemoradiotherapy was administered in the adjuvant setting, as two trials exhibited the ability to significantly reduce the local recurrence rate compared to treatment with surgery alone.[3,4] After the TME introduction a paradigm shift was introduced in preoperative radiotherapy. The Dutch TME trial demonstrated that neoadjuvant short course radiotherapy lead to a significant better local recurrence free survival.[5] The FFPOD 9203 and the EORTC 22921 trial both showed the benefits of concomitant chemotherapy alongside radiotherapy administered preoperatively in combination with TME surgery with regard to local recurrence rates.[6,7]

Theoretical background induction chemotherapy—advantages

Systemic effect

Treatment involving induction chemotherapy followed by neoadjuvant chemoradiotherapy, also referred to as total neoadjuvant treatment, has several theoretical advantages. Firstly, it is suggested that induction chemotherapy has the potential to eradicate micrometastasis. As mentioned, distant relapse remains a concern in patients with LARC with distant failure rates ranging between 20 and 30%. In the past, adjuvant chemotherapy was administered to diminish distant failure. In colon cancer, adjuvant chemotherapy improves survival for lymph node positive patients.

However, randomized trials assessing the value of adjuvant chemotherapy in patients with locally advanced rectal cancer have failed to demonstrate a significant benefit in disease free and overall survival.[8,9] The lack of survival benefit may be due to suboptimal compliance rates from poorly tolerated chemotherapy and long intervals between surgery and adjuvant chemotherapy. Induction chemotherapy has the potential to improve tolerability of therapy and addresses the inherent drawback of a long interval caused by postoperative morbidity.

Locoregional effect

Alongside the possible systemic advantage, addition of induction chemotherapy to the neoadjuvant treatment regimen may also improve local downstaging of the tumour. Biologically, solely the effect of induction chemotherapy could lead to improved local tumour downstaging. However, tumour shrinkage caused by induction chemotherapy could also potentially improve tumour vascularity, resulting in improved oxygenation and intratumoural levels of cytotoxic drugs, possibly enhancing tumour sensitivity to chemoradiotherapy and thereby increasing the locoregional effect of induction chemotherapy.[10] Clinically, improved local downstaging may improve resectability for initially unresectable tumours and help to achieve more R0 resections. Apart from the achievement of more R0 resections, improved local downstaging could also lead to a higher proportion of patients with a pathologic complete response (pCR). Alongside R0, pCR proved to be of prognostic value in predicting long-term outcome as patients with a pCR seem to have better long-term outcomes than those without pCR.[11–13]

Loco regional effect – conservative approach

Improved local downstaging may not only improve resectability of the tumour, it may also entail the possibility of more conservative surgery, such as sphincter preserving surgery. The addition of induction chemotherapy to the neoadjuvant treatment regimen may even result in more patients with a clinically complete response (cCR). In these patients with a clinical complete response a wait-and-see option could be considered since cCR is reported to have very low rates of both local recurrence and distant metastasis while also having an improved quality of life as well as improved functional outcomes in comparison to patients who underwent a TME resection.[14-16]

Assessment of tumour behaviour

Extending the neoadjuvant course by adding induction chemotherapy to the regimen provides an opportunity to assess the inherent tumour biological profile which allows timely identification of tumours with very aggressive natural behaviour, thereby omitting extensive surgery and subsequent morbidity.

Theoretical background induction chemotherapy—disadvantages

From a biological point of view, there have been concerns about the development of radioresistant cells in patients who fail to respond to chemotherapy, resulting in reduced efficacy of subsequent radiotherapy. Long-course induction chemotherapy may allow these drug-resistant clones to migrate to distant sites.[17] Clinically, the addition of induction chemotherapy may delay definitive chemoradiotherapy treatment due to chemotherapy-induced morbidity or reduce compliance to chemoradiotherapy. Moreover, this prolonged neoadjuvant treatment course may impact the performance status of patients who undergo planned surgical resection and thereby potentially increase surgical morbidity. Furthermore, delaying surgery because of chemotherapy induced morbidity may allow local disease progression, resulting in more challenging resections, increased morbidity, and even worse oncological outcomes.

Induction chemotherapy in locally advanced rectal cancer

Several RCTs, phase 2 trials and retrospective studies have been undertaken to study the effect of induction chemotherapy in LARC (Table 5.1). Chau et al. administered 3 cycles of CAPOX followed by chemoradiotherapy and TME surgery in 67 patients with MRI-defined poor-risk rectal cancer.[18] They observed an excellent R0 rate of 99%. They observed a pathological complete response in 16 patients (24%), which is promising when compared to the pCR rate after chemoradiotherapy alone (15-20%).[12] Koeberle at al.[19] conducted a single arm phase 2 study in 60 patients with T3-4 rectal cancer in whom they administered one cycle of CAPOX followed by radiotherapy with concomitant CAPOX. They reported similar outcomes to Chau et al. with a R0 resection rate of 98% and a pCR rate of 23%. However, in this study pCR was defined as a grade 3-4 according to the Dworak classification system, thereby including patients with near-complete regression in the pCR group. Complete tumour regression was observed in only seven patients (12%). Chua et al.[20] administered 4 cycles of CAPOX in 105 patients with MRI-defined poor-risk tumours and found a 22% pCR rate as well as an 98% R0 resection rate. They observed promising long-term results with an 86% 3-year disease-free survival (DFS) and a 83% overall survival (OS).

In contrast, Schou et al.,[21] who administered two cycles of CAPOX prior to chemoradiotherapy in 84 patients with LARC, described somewhat disappointing long-term results with a 5-year DFS and OS of 63% and 67% respectively despite a

Table 5.1 Overview of the literature regarding induction chemotherapy in patients with locally advanced rectal cancer

Study	Design	No.	Entry criteria	NAC regimen	CRT regimen	Adjuvant therapy	Compliance rate	pCR (%)	R0 (%)	Outcomes	Grade 3-4 toxicity	Clavien Dindo ≥3
Chau (2006)[31]	Cohort study Single arm	77	Poor-risk MRI features	CAPOX (3)	45Gy + capecitabine	Capecitabine (4)	91% NAC	24%	99%	1-year: - OS 95%	4 deaths	–
Chua[33] – Expert (2010)	Phase II Single arm	105	Poor-risk MRI features	CAPOX (4)	54Gy + capecitabine	CAPOX (4)	89% NAC; 91% RT	22%	98%	3-year: - DFS 86% - OS 83%	–	–
Golo[35]— OIGIT (2018)	Phase II Single arm	66	T2-4	Capecitabine (1) preRT—Capecitabine (2) postRT	45 Gy + capecitabine	Capecitabine (3)	- 99% RT - 86% Pre-nRT CT - 94% Post-nCRT CT	18%	98%	5-year: - DFS 64% - LRFS 93% - OS 70%	14%	–
Dewdney[44] (2012)	Phase II RCT	165	High-risk MRI features	CAPOX (4)	50.4Gy + capecitabine +/- cetuximab	CAPOX (4)	93% NAC; 90% RT	11%	92%	–	–	–
				CAPOX (4) + cetuximab	50.4Gy + capecitabine +/- cetuximab	CAPOX (4)	95% NAC; 91% RT	11%	96%			
Perez[39] – CONTRE(2017)	Phase II Single arm	39	T3-4 and/or N+	FOLFOX (6)	50.4Gy + capecitabine	None	92% NAC; 89% NAC+ RT	33%	–	After 25.5 m FU - LR 5.1% - DM 15%	–	–
Koeberle[32] (2008)	Phase II Single arm	60	T3-4	CAPOX (1)	45Gy + CAPOX	Left to treating physician discretion	93% RT	23%*	98%	–	–	–

Fernandez-Martos[45,46]—GCR-3 (2015)	Phase II RCT	108	T3-4	CAPOX (4)	50.4Gy + CAPOX	None	94% NAC; 85% RT	15%	89%	5-year - DFS 62% - OS 75% - LR 5% - DM 23%	19% NAC; 23% RT	51% (any grade)
					50.4Gy + CAPOX	CAPOX (4)	80% RT; 57% adj CT	15%	98%	- DFS 64% - OS 78% - LR 2% - DM 21%	54% adjCT; 29% RT	45% (any grade)
Maréchal[43] (2011)	Phase II RCT	57	T2-T4/N+	FOLFOX (2)	45Gy + 5-FU	None	97%	25%	86%	Closed due to futility	21% NAC; 7% RT	
					45Gy + 5-FU	None	96%	28%	96%		7% RT	
Schou[34] (2012)	Phase II Single arm	84	T3N+/MRF+T4	CAPOX (2)	54Gy + capecitabine	None	–	25%	94%	5-year: - DFS 63% - OS 67%	18% NAC (+ 4 death); 11% RT	21%
Tang[40] (2018)	Prospective cohort study	45		CAPOX (1) postRT	50Gy + CAPOX (2 cycles)	CAPOX (5)		38%	100%	3year - DFS 76% - OS 89%		
Calvo[42] (2014)	Non-randomized Two arms	335	T3-4 and/or N+	FOLFOX (2)	50.4Gy + 5-FU/tegafur	5-FU (4–6)	–	–	96%	- T downstaging 63% - N downstaging 60% - Sphincter sparing 30% - LR 7% - 10-year DFS 72%	29%	25%

(*continued*)

Table 5.1 Continued

Study	Design	No.	Entry criteria	NAC regimen	CRT regimen	Adjuvant therapy	Compliance rate	pCR (%)	R0 (%)	Outcomes	Grade 3-4 toxicity	Clavien Dindo ≥3
					50.4Gy + 5-FU/tegafur	5-FU (4–6)	–	–	97%	- T downstaging 54% - N downstaging 43% - Sphincter sparing 13% - LR 9% - 10-year DFS 68%	33%	22%
Garcia-Aguilar[37] (2015)	Phase II Four arms Non-randomized	259	T2-4/N+		50.4Gy + 5-FU	None		18%	98%	- Sphincter saving: 77%/75%/75%/68%	29% CRT (all groups)	15%
				FOLFOX (2)	50.4Gy + 5-FU	None	82% NAC	25%	100%		4% NAC	6%
				FLOFOX (4)	50.4Gy + 5-FU	None	81% NAC	30%	96%		18% NAC	4%
				FOLFOX (6)	50.4Gy + 5-FU	None	77% NAC	38%	100%		35% NAC	9%
Nogue[38] (2011)	Phase II Single arm	47	T3-4	CAPOX (4) + bevacuzimab	50.4Gy + bevacuzimab	None	–	36%	98%		2 deaths	58% (any grade)
Wang[36] (2018)	Phase II Single arm	47	High-risk MRI features	CAPOX (3) preRT - CAPOX (3) postRT	50.4Gy + CAPOX	None	98% RT; 72% NAC	30% pCR; 6% cCR	100%	–	–	–

Hu[41] (2018)	Phase II Single arm	49	High-risk MRI features	CAPOX (1) preRT—CAPOX (1) postRT	50Gy + CAPOX (2)	None	–	42%	100%	5-year: - OS 91% - DFS 80% - DM 20% - LR 2%	–	–
Cercek[47] (2018)	Retrospective cohort Two arms	628	T3-4 and/or N+	FOLFOX (8)/ CAPOX (5) / FLOX	50.4 Gy + 5-FU/ capecitabine	None	96% 5-FU, 90% oxaliplatin	18% pCR; 22% cCR	–	–	–	–
					50.4 Gy + 5-FU/ capecitabine	FOLFOX/ CAPOX/ FLOX	88% 5-FU, 73% oxaliplatin	17% pCR; 6% cCR	–	–	–	–

No. number; NAC, neoadjuvant chemotherapy; CRT, chemoradiotherapy; pCR, pathologic complete response; R0, resection with clear resection margins (N) number of chemotherapy cycles; CAPOX (capecitabine + oxaliplatin); FOLFOX (5-fluorouracil + leucovorin + oxaliplatin); FLOX (5-fluorouracil + leucovorin + oxaliplatin)5FU 5-fluorouracil; RT radiotherapy; OS overall survival; DFS; DM distant metastasis rate; LR local recurrence rate* defined as Dworak grading 3–4.

25% pCR rate and a 94% R0 resection rate. Golo et al used induction chemotherapy consisting of one cycle of capecitabine prior to radiotherapy with concomitant capecitabine.[22] In the resting time between chemoradiotherapy and surgery another cycle of capecitabine was administered. In the 66 patients enrolled in this study pCR rate was rather disappointing (18%). However, R0 resection rate was still 98% and long-term results were comparable with results from Schou et al., as five-year DFS and OS were 64% and 70% respectively.

More encouraging pCR rates are reported in studies by Wang,[23] Garcia,[24] and Nogue.[25] Wang et al.[23] conducted a single arm phase II trial in which they administered three cycles CAPOX prior to radiotherapy with concomitant CAPOX followed by another three cycles of CAPOX in 47 patients. In 30% of patients a pCR was achieved and all patients underwent a R0 resection. Clinical complete response was seen in 6% of patients. Despite this intensified treatment regimen, no grade 4 or 5 toxicities were observed and major surgical complications were treated conservatively. Nogue et al.[25] added bevacuzimab to induction chemotherapy with CAPOX in 47 patients, resulting in a very high pCR rate of 36% and a 98% R0 resection rate. However, two patients died during induction chemotherapy.

Garcia-Aguilar et al.[24] designed a regimen wherein chemotherapy was delivered after chemoradiotherapy. In a total of 259 patients they compared four different treatment arms with intensifying chemotherapy regimen and observed that six cycles of FOLFOX administered after chemoradiotherapy translated into a significant better pCR rate (38%) compared to treatment without, with two or with four cycles of chemotherapy (18%, 25%, 30% respectively). Despite this significant difference in pCR rate, R0 resection rates were comparable for all four groups (98%, 100%, 96%, 100% respectively). The proportion of patients experiencing grade 3-4 toxicity increased with increasing number of cycles, up to 35% in patients receiving six cycles of chemotherapy.

Perez[26], Tang,[27] and Hu[28] did report on long-term results in their studies. In the CONTRE study by Perez et al. induction chemotherapy consisted of six cycles of FOLFOX. They observed a high pCR of 33% and a distant metastasis rate of only 15%. However, median follow-up was only 25 months. Tang et al. administered one cycle of CAPOX after radiotherapy treatment with two concomitant cycles of CAPOX. Adjuvant treatment consisted of five cycles of CAPOX. They demonstrated a 38% pCR rate and a R0 resection rate of 100%. Oncological outcomes were promising with a 3-year OS of 89% and a 76% DFS. Treatment regimen in the study conducted by Hu et al. consisted of one cycle of CAPOX administered prior chemoradiotherapy and one cycle post-radiotherapy. No adjuvant therapy was prescribed. Five-year overall and disease free survival were 91% and 80% respectively and cumulative incidence of distant metastasis was 20% after a median follow-up of 60 months. Despite these promising long-term results in several smaller studies, one large non-randomized study performed in 335 patients comparing treatment with induction chemotherapy (2 cycles FOLFOX) followed by chemoradiotherapy with concomitant 5-FU and adjuvant chemotherapy versus treatment without induction chemotherapy did not find any different between the two treatment arms. R0 resection rates were 96% and 97% respectively and DFS was 72% versus 68% after 10 years.[29]

Three randomized trials failed to demonstrate improved pCR and R0 rates for patient treated with induction chemotherapy. The smallest of three studies, including 57 patients, administered 2 cycles of FOLFOX as induction chemotherapy followed by chemoradiotherapy.[30] Despite the promising pCR rate of 25% in patient treated with FOLFOX, patients in the non-induction chemotherapy arm had a 28% pCR rate. R0 resection rates were 96% and 86% for the induction and non-induction chemotherapy arm respectively. In the randomized study by Dewdney et al.[31] induction chemotherapy consisted of either four cycles CAPOX or four cycles CAPOX with cetuximab. Subsequently both study arms received radiotherapy with concomitant capecitabine with or without cetuximab and adjuvant therapy consisted of four cycles CAPOX. Observed pCR rates were disappointing; 7% and 11%, respectively. The third randomized trial including 108 patients compared induction chemotherapy followed by chemoradiotherapy with chemoradiotherapy and adjuvant chemotherapy.[32,33] Both induction and adjuvant chemotherapy consisted of four cycles of CAPOX. Despite significant difference in compliance rates to chemotherapy (94% vs. 57% respectively), outcomes were comparable. pCR rate were 15% for both treatment arms and R0 resection rates were 89% and 98%. Five-year outcomes were not favourable for the induction chemotherapy arm. DFS was 62% vs. 64% and OS was 75% vs. 78%, respectively.

Despite the poor results in these randomized trials, a recent RCT and a network meta-analysis have showed promising results for total neoadjuvant therapy. The PRODIGE 23 trial randomly assigned 461 patients to either neoadjuvant chemotherapy group (FOLFIRINOX, CRT, TME, and adjuvant therapy) or standard therapy (CRT, TME, and adjuvant therapy).[34] The pCR rate was significantly better in the neoadjuvant chemotherapy group (27.5% vs. 11.7%) with a lower local relapse seen in this group also (4.8% vs. 7%). Both three-year DFS (75.5% vs. 68.5%) and OS (90.8% vs. 87.7%) were better in the neoadjuvant chemotherapy group. A network meta-analysis on randomized control trials conducted by Donnelly et al has further added support to total neoadjuvant therapy. Fifteen RCTs were included in the analysis, with total neoadjuvant therapy showing improved OS, rates of distant metastasis, and reduced overall recurrences. Both a cCR and pCR were improved in the total neoadjuvant group, however, no difference was seen in DFS, local recurrence, RO resection rates, compliance, or toxicity.[35]

Organ preservation and total neoadjuvant therapy

A large retrospective study reporting on outcomes of induction chemotherapy in patients with LARC described interesting results regarding clinical complete response. A total of 628 patients received either FOLFOX, CAPOX, or FLOX followed by chemoradiotherapy or chemoradiotherapy alone. pCR rates in both treatment arms were comparable (18% vs. 17% respectively). However, another 22% of patients in the induction chemotherapy treatment arm had a sustained clinical complete response and did not undergo surgery. This was significantly better compared to patients treated with chemoradiotherapy alone, in whom only 6% had a sustained clinical complete response (cCR). While long-term follow-up in this cohort is not available yet, but the conclusion may be that total neoadjuvant facilitates nonoperative treatment strategies in patients with LARC. This has been shown however in the recent randomized OPRA trial. This phase II trial enrolled 324 patients into induction chemotherapy followed by CRT or CRT and consolidation chemotherapy followed by TME or watch and wait. The three-year DFS was 76% in both groups, with three-year TME free survival of 41% in the induction group and 53% in the consolidation group. No difference was seen in local recurrence-free survival, distant metastasis, or OS. This highlights that total neoadjuvant therapy can achieve organ preservation in half of patients without a detrimental impact on oncological outcomes.[37] Furthermore, the German CAO/ARO/AIO-12 trial randomly assigned patients to receive either induction or consolidation chemotherapy. They noted a higher compliance rate in the consolidation chemotherapy group, with an improved pCR also seen in this group (25% vs. 17%). Three-year DFS was similar between the groups, along with the three-year cumulative incidence of locoregional recurrence and distant metastasis. They favoured using consolidation chemotherapy as the preferred route if organ preservation is the goal of treatment.[38]

Limitations to the literature

Altogether, the results from the addition of induction chemotherapy to the neoadjuvant treatment of patients with LARC vary widely when comparing pCR and R0 resection rates and long-term results are either lacking or are contradictory. This could be due to the considerable heterogeneity in selection of patients, in initial staging, in the cytotoxic and biological drugs used in the neoadjuvant treatment regimen and the timing, duration, and dose intensity of the induction chemotherapy. In addition, the radiotherapy component varied in total dose and fraction size when comparing the different studies. These sometimes discouraging results could not be the result of poor compliance to total neoadjuvant treatment as compliance rates in all studies were high (80–100%). As demonstrated by Fernandez et al.[32] this is much higher compared to when chemotherapy is administered in the adjuvant setting. In addition, administration of induction chemotherapy did not seem to delay or influence compliance rates to chemoradiotherapy. In the aforementioned studies, 3–11% of patients dropped out during neoadjuvant treatment and did not undergo surgery. Reported details on why patients did not undergo surgery were the development of distant metastasis, comorbidity, or worsened performance status due to the administration of neoadjuvant treatment, refusal of surgery by the patient or death related to the infusion of induction chemotherapy. Although the dropout percentage in these studies is low despite a fairly intensive neoadjuvant treatment regimen, it should be noted that in the majority of the studies only relatively fit patients were included.

The reported toxicity of the total neoadjuvant treatment strategy varies. Some studies reported relatively low percentages of patients with grade 3–4 toxicities, whereas others reported several deaths related to the infusion of induction chemotherapy. This variation could again be caused by the different chemotherapy agents used in the neoadjuvant treatment regimen, as well as the differences in timing, duration, and intensity. Whether the addition of induction chemotherapy to the treatment of LARC will be the solution to reduce distant metastasis and improve oncological outcomes remains to be elucidated

Conclusion

From a theoretical point of view, total neoadjuvant treatment seems a logical step to improve surgical and oncological outcomes. Based on retrospective research, the addition of induction chemotherapy seems feasible with high compliance rates, without compromising the ability to undergo chemoradiotherapy and surgery, with moderate toxicity and acceptable postoperative morbidity. However, the results for the addition of induction chemotherapy to the neoadjuvant treatment of LARC vary widely when comparing R0 resection and pCR rates and the impact on overall and local recurrence free survival is unclear. Perhaps the most important innovation will be the increasing rate of clinical complete responses, making it possible to omit radical surgery in patients in whom surgery has always been the cornerstone of treatment.

References

1. Heald RJ, Moran BJ, Ryall RDH, Sexton R, Macfarlane JK. Rectal cancer: the Basingstoke experience of total mesorectal excision, 1978–1997. *Arch Surg.* 1998;133:894–9.
2. Wibe A, Møller B, Norstein J, et al. A national strategic change in treatment policy for rectal cancer—implementation of total mesorectal excision as routine treatment in Norway. A national audit. *Dis Colon Rectum.* 2002;45(7):857–66.
3. Krook JE, Collins RT, Kubista TP, et al. Effective surgical adjuvant therapy for high-risk rectal carcinoma. *N Engl J Med.* 1991;324(11):709–15.
4. Gastrointestinal Tumor Study Group. Radiation therapy and fluorouracil with or without semustine for the treatment of patients with surgical adjuvant adenocarcinoma of the rectum. *J Clin Oncol.* 1992;10(4):549–57.
5. Kapiteijn E, Marijnen CAM, Nagtegaal ID, et al. Preoperative radiotherapy combined with total mesorectal excision for resectable rectal cancer. *N Engl J Med.* 2001;345(9):638–46.
6. Gérard JP, Conroy T, Bonnetain F, et al. Preoperative radiotherapy with or without concurrent fluorouracil and leucovorin in T3-4 rectal cancers: Results of FFCD 9203. *J Clin Oncol.* 2006;24(28):4620–5.
7. Bosset JF, Collette L, Calais G, et al. Chemotherapy with preoperative radiotherapy in rectal cancer. *N Engl J Med.* 2006;355(11):1114–23.

8. Collette L, Bosset JF, Den Dulk M, et al. Patients with curative resection of cT3–4 rectal cancer after preoperative radiotherapy or radiochemotherapy: does anybody benefit from adjuvant fluorouracil-based chemotherapy? A trial of the European Organisation for Research and Treatment of Cancer Radiation Oncology Group. *J Clin Oncol.* 2007;25(28):4379–86.
9. Breugom AJ, Van Gijn W, Muller EW, et al. Adjuvant chemotherapy for rectal cancer patients treated with preoperative (chemo)radiotherapy and total mesorectal excision: a Dutch Colorectal Cancer Group (DCCG) randomized phase III trial. *Ann Oncol.* 2015;26(4):696–701.
10. Milas L, Hunter NR, Mason KA, Milross CG, Saito Y, Peters LJ. Role of reoxygenation in induction of enhancement of tumor radioresponse by paclitaxel. *Cancer Res.* 1995;55(16):3564–8.
11. Kong JC, Guerra GR, Warrier SK, et al. Prognostic value of tumour regression grade in locally advanced rectal cancer: a systematic review and meta-analysis. *Color Dis.* 2018;20(7):574–85.
12. Maas M, Nelemans J, Marañón G, et al. Long-term outcome in patients with a pathological complete response after chemoradiation for rectal cancer: a pooled analysis of individual patient data. *Lancet Oncol.* 2010;11:835–79.
13. Martin ST, Heneghan HM, Winter DC. Systematic review and meta-analysis of outcomes following pathological complete response to neoadjuvant chemoradiotherapy for rectal cancer. *Br J Surg.* 2012;99:918–28.
14. Maas M, Beets-Tan RGH, Lambregts DMJ, et al. Wait-and-see policy for clinical complete responders after chemoradiation for rectal cancer. *J Clin Oncol.* 2011; 29(35):4633–40.
15. Hupkens BJP, Martens MH, Stoot JH, et al. Quality of life in rectal cancer patients after chemoradiation: watch-and-wait policy versus standard resection—matched-controlled study. *Dis Colon Rectum.* 2017;60(10):1032–40.
16. van der Valk MJM, Hilling DE, Bastiaannet E, et al. Long-term outcomes of clinical complete responders after neoadjuvant treatment for rectal cancer in the International Watch & Wait Database (IWWD): an international multicentre registry study. *Lancet.* 2018;391(10139):2537–45.
17. Glynne-Jones R, Grainger J, Harrison M, Ostler P, Makris A. Neoadjuvant chemotherapy prior to preoperative chemoradiation or radiation in rectal cancer: Should we be more cautious? *Br J Cancer.* 2006;94(3):363–71.
18. Chau I, Brown G, Cunningham D, et al. Neoadjuvant capecitabine and oxaliplatin followed by synchronous chemoradiation and total mesorectal excision in magnetic resonance imaging-defined poor-risk rectal cancer. *J Clin Oncol.* 2006;24(4):668–74.
19. Koeberle D, Burkhard R, Von Moos R, et al. Phase II study of capecitabine and oxaliplatin given prior to and concurrently with preoperative pelvic radiotherapy in patients with locally advanced rectal cancer. *Br J Cancer.* 2008;98(7):1204–9.
20. Chua YJ, Barbachano Y, Cunningham D, et al. Neoadjuvant capecitabine and oxaliplatin before chemoradiotherapy and total mesorectal excision in MRI-defined poor-risk rectal cancer: a phase 2 trial. *Lancet Oncol.* 2010;11(3):241–8.
21. Schou J V., Larsen FO, Rasch L, et al. Induction chemotherapy with capecitabine and oxaliplatin followed by chemoradiotherapy before total mesorectal excision in patients with locally advanced rectal cancer. *Ann Oncol.* 2012;23(10):2627–33.
22. Golo D, But-Hadzic J, Anderluh F, et al. Induction chemotherapy, chemoradiotherapy and consolidation chemotherapy in preoperative treatment of rectal cancer—long-term results of phase II OIGIT-01 Trial. *Radiol Oncol.* 2018;52(3):267–74.
23. Wang X, Yu Y, Meng W, et al. Total neoadjuvant treatment (CAPOX plus radiotherapy) for patients with locally advanced rectal cancer with high risk factors: A phase 2 trial. *Radiother Oncol.* 2018;129(2):300–5.

24. Garcia-Aguilar J, Chow OS, Smith DD, et al. Effect of adding mFOLFOX6 after neoadjuvant chemoradiation in locally advanced rectal cancer: a multicentre, phase 2 trial. *Lancet Oncol.* 2015;16(8):957–66.
25. Nogue M, Salud A, Vicente P, et al. Addition of bevacizumab to XELOX induction therapy plus concomitant capecitabine-based chemoradiotherapy in magnetic resonance imaging-defined poor-prognosis locally advanced rectal cancer: the AVACROSS study. *Oncologist.* 2011;16(5):614–20.
26. Perez K, Safran H, Sikov W, et al. Complete neoadjuvant treatment for rectal cancer: The Brown University Oncology Group CONTRE study. *Am J Clin Oncol Cancer Clin Trials.* 2017;40(3):283–7.
27. Tang J, Wu X, Bai Y, et al. Long-term outcome of oxaliplatin and capecitabine (XELOX) concomitant with neoadjuvant radiotherapy and extended to the resting period in high risk locally advanced rectal cancer. *J Cancer.* 2018;9(8):1365–70.
28. Hu YH, Wei JW, Chang H, et al. The high pCR rate of sandwich neoadjuvant treatment in locally advanced rectal cancer may translate into a better long-term survival benefit: 5-year outcome of a phase II clinical trial. *Cancer Manag Res.* 2018;10:4363–9.
29. Calvo FA, Sole C V., Serrano J, et al. Preoperative chemoradiation with or without induction oxaliplatin plus 5-fluorouracil in locally advanced rectal cancer: long-term outcome analysis. *Strahlentherapie und Onkol.* 2014;190(2):149–57.
30. Maréchal R, Vos B, Polus M, et al. Short course chemotherapy followed by concomitant chemoradiotherapy and surgery in locally advanced rectal cancer: a randomized multicentric phase II study. *Ann Oncol.* 2012;23(6):1525–30.
31. Dewdney A, Cunningham D, Tabernero J, et al. Multicenter randomized phase II clinical trial comparing neoadjuvant oxaliplatin, capecitabine, and preoperative radiotherapy with or without cetuximab followed by total mesorectal excision in patients with high-risk rectal cancer (EXPERT-C). *J Clin Oncol.* 2012;30(14):1620–7.
32. Fernández-Martos C, Pericay C, Aparicio J, et al. Phase II, randomized study of concomitant chemoradiotherapy followed by surgery and adjuvant capecitabine plus oxaliplatin (CAPOX) compared with induction CAPOX followed by concomitant chemoradiotherapy and surgery in magnetic resonance imaging-defined, l. *J Clin Oncol.* 2010;28(5):859–65.
33. Fernández-Martos C, Garcia-Albeniz X, Pericay C, et al. Chemoradiation, surgery and adjuvant chemotherapy versus induction chemotherapy followed by chemoradiation and surgery: long-term results of the Spanish GCR-3 phase II randomized trial. *Ann Oncol.* 2015;26(8):1722–8.
34. Conroy T, Bosset JF et al. Neoadjuvant chemotherapy with FOLFIRINOX and preoperative chemoradiotherapy for patients with locally advanced rectal cancer (UNICANCER-PRODIGE 23): a multicentre, randomised, open-label, phase 3 trial. *Lancet Oncol.* 2021;22(5):702–15.
35. Donnelly M et al. Total neodajuvant therapy versus standard neoadjuvant treatment strategies for the management of locally advanced rectal cancer: network meta-analysis of randomized clinical trials. *BJS.* 2023:110:1316–30.
36. Cercek A, Roxburgh CSD, Strombom P, et al. Adoption of total neoadjuvant therapy for locally advanced rectal cancer. *JAMA Oncol.* 2018;4(6):e180071.
37. Garcia-Aguilar J, Patil S, Gollub MJ, et al. Organ preservation in patients with rectal adenocarcinoma treated with total neoadjuvant therapy. *J Clin Oncol.* 2022;40(23):2546–56.
38. Fokas E, Schlenska-Lange A, Polat B, et al. Chemoradiotherapy plus induction or consolidation chemotherapy as total neoadjuvant therapy for patients with locally advanced rectal cancer: long-term results of the CAO/ARO/AIO-12 randomized clinical trial. *JAMA Oncol.* 2022;8(1):e215445.

6

Watch and wait in locally advanced rectal cancer

Ishwarya Balasubramanian, Ben Creavin, and Desmond Winter

Introduction

Neoadjuvant chemoradiotherapy (NACRT) induces downstaging in rectal cancer, with cCR seen in 10–30% of patients.[1] In patients with cCR, the standard total mesorectal (TME) excision (anterior resection or abdominoperineal resection) can be avoided, which is associated with 1–2% of perioperative mortality that increases with old age, frailty, and comorbidities.[2] Instead, organ preservation strategies can be offered, which include local excision through the anus or conservative management without resection. The latter has gained increasing interest since being first described in 2004 by Habr-Gama and Colleagues and introduces the concept of 'watch and wait' through active surveillance in rectal cancer patients who had achieved cCR following NACRT.[3] This approach spares patients from complications associated with rectal resection, including urinary and sexual dysfunction, faecal incontinence, and associated high rates of permanent stoma.

The watch and wait surveillance follows a three-pillar assessment, which includes[4]

1. Digital rectal examination—smooth surface of the rectal wall without palpable induration, ulceration, irregularities, or stenosis of the rectum.
2. Endoscopic assessment—white scar without evidence of ulceration of the rectal wall or mucosal irregularities on flexible endoscopy, which can be further clarified on narrow band imaging.
3. Radiological imaging—assessment of the mesorectum and lateral pelvic compartment for the presence of residual disease within lymph nodes, vascular structures, and tumour deposits reported using the MRI tumour regression grade classification.

Interestingly, endoscopic biopsies post-NACRT are not routinely used in diagnosing cCR. This is due to the low negative predictive value of 21% as a diagnostic tool; therefore, a negative endoscopic biopsy is not predictive of an incomplete clinical response to avoid a radical resection.[5] Rectal cancer patients who achieve cCR as per these strict clinical, endoscopic, and radiological criteria may benefit from organ preservation strategies. These patients need to be enrolled in a close surveillance programme that comprises these three pillars to ensure early detection of tumour regrowth and distant metastases.

Safety of watch and wait—Brazilian experience

In the initial study reported by Habr-Gama and colleagues, surveillance consisted of monthly digital rectal examination, proctoscopy +/– biopsies, 6 monthly CT scans of chest, abdomen, and pelvis, and carcinoembryonic antigen (CEA) levels in year 1. This was then stretched out to 2 months in year 2 and 6 months in year 3. Furthermore, it showed no difference in overall survival (100% vs. 97%) or disease-free survival (86% vs. 84%) between operative and watch and wait at 10 years of follow-up.[3]

These results were further validated in a follow-up of 99 patients who sustained cCR for at least 12 months and were considered as clinical stage 0. cCR is defined as the absence of residual mass, ulcer, or suspicious scar clinically and endoscopically, with no signs of residual tumour seen in radiological studies at 8 weeks following NACRT. The overall survival and disease-free survival at five years in this cohort were 93% and 85%, respectively. Of the 13.1% recurrences observed in this cohort, 5 were endorectal, 7 systemic, and 1 combined recurrences.[6] They hypothesized that the majority of recurrences were systemic failures due to occult disseminated microscopic foci undetectable by standard radiological assessment as opposed to local recurrences, which is a concern in the uptake of this approach. Local recurrences in this cohort were significantly associated with radiological evidence of positive lymph nodes ($p = 0.03$) and stage cIII ($p = 0.01$). [6] In addition, it is reported that the local recurrence occurs late in comparison to distant recurrence (mean recurrence interval 52 ± 23.1 vs. 29.5 ± 26.9 months) and is frequently amenable to salvage surgery, resulting in excellent long-term survival rates. It is important to distinguish this from recurrences encountered following TME surgery, which is associated with poor outcomes and often unresectable. Hence, many refer to recurrences following NACRT as regrowth to avoid the concern associated with the latter surgical approach.[7]

Furthermore, the recent advances in neoadjuvant regimes have supported low local recurrence rates, even in those with initial node-positive disease. Habr-Gama et al. found no difference in surgery-free survival (39.7% vs. 46.8%, $p = 0.2$) and distant metastases-free survival (77.5% vs. 80.5%, $p = 0.49$) at five years between node-positive and node-negative patients. Hence, they concluded that initial node-positive disease followed by cCR after NACRT is not associated with increased risk of tumour recurrence or development of more advanced disease at the time of recurrence.[8,9] Thus, it was advocated that a nonoperative approach with watch-and-wait surveillance is safe, and associated with good survival rates in highly selective patients who achieved cCR.[6,8,9]

Safety of watch and wait—international experience

Maas et al. identified 21 patients with cCR following a chemoradiotherapy (CRT) regimen of capecitabine and 50.4 Gy radiotherapy. Definition of cCR was stricter in this study, with assessment of cCR based on endoscopic and radiological modalities: (i) No residual tumour on MRI with the presence of fibrosis only; (ii) absence of suspicious lymph node on MRI; (iii) only residual ulcer or scar at endoscopy; (iv) negative biopsy samples from the scar, ulcer, or prior tumour location; and (v) no palpable lesion on DRE.[10] Local recurrence occurred in 1 patient in the 'watch-and-wait' group at 22 months. Overall survival and disease-free survival were 100% and 89% in the 'watch-and-wait' group compared to 91% and 93% in the control group (surgical resection following neoadjuvant therapy), respectively.[10]

The Oncological Outcomes after Clinical Complete Response in Patients with Rectal Cancer (OnCoRe) group developed one-to-one paired cohorts of watch and wait versus surgical resection patients using propensity-score matching (T stage, age, and performance status).[11] In total, 129 patients were treated with a 'watch-and-wait' approach, of which local recurrences occurred in 34% of patients at three years. Salvage resection was successful in 88% of these patients. There was no difference in three-year non-regrowth disease-free survival or three-year overall survival (96% vs. 87%, $p = 0.043$). They noted a 26% absolute difference in avoidance of a permanent stoma at three years.[11]

Smith et al. managed 32 patients conservatively with wait-and-wait approach following cCR. Non-operative management was associated with lower pretreatment stage, old age, and distal tumour location ($p < 0.05$). There was no difference in the 2-year distance-free survival (88% vs. 98%, $p = 0.27$) and overall survival (96% vs. 100%, $p = 0.56$) between the watch-and-wait and resection groups. In the watch-and-wait group, six patients had local recurrence, of whom three went on to develop concurrent distant recurrences. All six patients were managed by salvage rectal resection with no further recurrence of disease at a median follow-up of 17 months. The author concluded that watch-and-wait surveillance achieves similar local and distant disease control compared with patients with cCR undergoing rectal resections.[12]

With the use of the American Veterans Administration Central Cancer registry, Spiegel et al. explored the role of watch and wait in locally advanced rectal cancer. Of the 1,313 patients identified, 20.8% of 313 patients who underwent NACRT alone and 10.5% of 1,000 patients who underwent NACRT followed by surgery had cCR. They reported similar median overall survival ($p = 0.128$) and disease-specific survival ($p = 0.161$) between NACRT and NACRT followed by surgery.[13]

Dossa et al. performed a pooled analysis of 867 patients from 23 studies, with a median follow-up of 12–68 months. The majority of patients included were male and aged between 39 and 86 years. The watch-and-wait approach in this cohort was commonly undertaken in high-risk surgical patients or based on patients' preference following discussion with their surgeon. This study reported a two-year local regrowth rate of 15.7% with the majority of these patients (95.4%) undergoing salvage treatment. No significant difference in non-regrowth recurrence or cancer-specific mortality was seen between patients managed with watch and wait after cCR and patients with pathological complete response at resection.[14]

Dattani et al. performed a meta-analysis assessing the role of watch and wait in rectal cancer. Using 17 studies, they showed a cCR of 22.4% with a local regrowth rate of 22.1% within the first three years. Salvage surgery was performed in 88% with R0 resection rates of 93%. Three-year overall survival was 93.5%. They concluded that watch and wait is a safe approach; however, robust surveillance is required.[15]

The International Watch and Wait Database (IWWD)

This is the largest multicentre observational registry study that reports on pooled individual patient data with rectal cancer and cCR after neoadjuvant therapy, treated with a watch-and-wait strategy internationally. Van der Valk et al. reported in the first series on 880 patients from 47 centres across 15 countries. This study echoed the safety of watch and wait with excellent five-year overall survival rates of 84.7% and five-year disease-specific survival rates of 93.8%. The cumulative incidence of local recurrence was 25% with 88% of these occurring within the first two years. The majority of re-growths (97%) were located in the bowel wall and managed successfully with curative intent.[16]

Fernandez et al. added clarity to the safety of this approach and the level of surveillance required in patients being managed by watch-and-wait surveillance. Regrowth-free survival estimates of patients who had sustained cCR for 3, 5, and 7 years were high at 88.1%, 97.3%, and 98.6%, respectively. Similar high rates of 93.8%, 97.8%, and 96.6% are observed for distant metastasis-free survival. Hence, they report that the risks for local growth and distant metastases during the subsequent two years are notably low, thus reducing the intensity of active surveillance after the initial three years of starting this approach.[17] However, it has been shown that patients who do develop local regrowth are at higher risk for development of distant metastases compared to patients without local regrowth (five-year conditional distant metastases-free survival 94.9% vs. 98.4%).[18]

Previous studies have reported that although younger patients are diagnosed with more advanced-stage disease, these patients were more likely to be treated with long-course NACRT and hence achieve cCR.[19,20] However, concerns remain regarding whether this approach would be oncologically safe in patients with young-onset cancer. Bearing this in mind, IWWD analysed outcomes of watch and wait in 199 rectal cancer patients to see if this was a feasible option in patients aged less than 50 years. Bahadoer et al. reported no difference in disease-specific survival rate at three years between patients aged below 50 years and those aged over 50 years (98% vs. 97%). Further to this, no difference in local regrowth rates at three years was seen between the two groups (24% vs. 26%). They recommended a shared decision-making process with younger patients who achieved cCR after NACRT, when offering watch and wait in dedicated centres with careful risk assessments and surveillance programmes.[19]

The future of watch and wait

Improving response rates to neoadjuvant therapy is the key to offering organ preservation to more patients. Therefore, the use of total neoadjuvant therapy has become popular to improve both oncological outcomes and organ preservation management. The Organ Preservation in patients with Rectal Adenocarcinoma treated with total neoadjuvant therapy (OPRA) trial is a randomized phase II trial that assessed the outcomes of 324 patients with stage II/III rectal cancer treated with induction chemotherapy followed by chemoradiotherapy or chemoradiotherapy followed by consolidation chemotherapy and either TME or watch-and-wait surveillance based on the basis of tumour response. Although the three-year disease-free survival was similar at 76% in both groups, the three-year TME-free survival was 41% and 53% for induction chemotherapy and consolidation chemotherapy, respectively. Garcia-Aguillar et al. concluded that the sequence of chemotherapy in total neoadjuvant chemotherapy did not affect disease-free survival, but a higher rate of organ preservation was observed in induction chemotherapy followed by chemoradiotherapy.[21] The PRODIGE23 trial also showed promising oncological and complete response rates in patients undergoing total neoadjuvant therapy. Complete response rates were double in the total neoadjuvant group (28% vs. 12%), and 3-year disease-free survival was also better in this group compared to standard neoadjuvant therapy (76% vs. 69%).[22] Furthermore, the CAO/ARO/AIO-12 trial again showed improved pathological complete response rates (25% vs. 17%) in patients receiving total neoadjuvant therapy.[23] These studies highlight the increasing role total neoadjuvant therapy has on complete response rates and the increasing possibility that more patients may be treated with organ preservation with these approaches. However, consensus on the exact total neoadjuvant regime is still lacking.

Although a small number of rectal cancers are mismatch repair-deficient (5–10%), recent reports on the use of immunotherapy in this cohort have shown excellent results. A recent report in the *New England Journal of Medicine* assessed PDL-1 Blockade in 12 mismatch-deficient rectal cancers. All patients achieved a complete clinical response to therapy without the need for standard chemoradiotherapy or surgery. Furthermore, no recurrences were observed at 25 months.[24] Although these results need to be interpreted cautiously due to low numbers and short follow-up, it is a promising approach for mismatch-deficient rectal cancers that could achieve a complete response without the adverse effects of chemoradiotherapy and surgery.

Summary

The role of radical surgery with the associated potential for significant morbidity has been challenged in patients with cCR. Instead of assessing cCR with a watch-and-wait surveillance through clinical, endoscopic, and radiological investigations has become a feasible approach in rectal cancer patients downstaged following NACRT. Although the uptake has been slow, a greater willingness to adopt a watch-and-wait strategy has been shown as more focus is given to patient-reported outcomes.[25] Although randomized controlled trials are lacking, the published studies to date and data so far from the International Watch and Wait database provide evidence to support the safety and feasibility of watch-and-wait surveillance. However, further research is required to standardize the definitions of cCR, chemoradiotherapy regimens, surveillance protocols, and outcomes reported from centres undertaking watch-and-wait surveillance.

References

1. Martin ST, Heneghan HM, Winter DC. Systematic review and meta-analysis of outcomes following pathological complete response to neoadjuvant chemoradiotherapy for rectal cancer. *Br J Surg*. Jul 2012;99(7):918–28.
2. Teste B, Rouanet P, Tuech JJ, et al. Early and late morbidity of local excision after chemoradiotherapy for rectal cancer. *BJS Open*. 2021;5(3):zrab043.
3. Habr-Gama A, Perez RO, Nadalin W, et al. Operative versus nonoperative treatment for stage 0 distal rectal cancer following chemoradiation therapy: long-term results. *Ann Surg*. 2004;240(4):711–17; discussion 717–18.
4. Cerdan-Santacruz C, São Julião GP, Vailati BB, Corbi L, Habr-Gama A, Perez RO. Watch and wait approach for rectal cancer. *J Clin Med*. 2023;12(8):2873.
5. Perez RO, Habr-Gama A, Pereira GV, et al. Role of biopsies in patients with residual rectal cancer following neoadjuvant chemoradiation after downsizing: can they rule out persisting cancer? *Colorectal Dis*. 2012;14(6):714–20.
6. Habr-Gama A, Perez RO, Proscurshim I, et al. Patterns of failure and survival for nonoperative treatment of stage c0 distal rectal cancer following neoadjuvant chemoradiation therapy. *J Gastrointest Surg*. 2006;10(10):1319–28; discussion 1328–9.
7. Heald RJ, Beets G, Carvalho C. Report from a consensus meeting: response to chemoradiotherapy in rectal cancer—predictor of cure and a crucial new choice for the patient. *Colorectal Dis*. 2014;16(5):334–7.
8. Habr-Gama A, São Julião GP, Vailati BB, et al. Organ preservation among patients with clinically node-positive rectal cancer: is it really more dangerous? *Dis Colon Rectum*. 2019;62(6):675–83.
9. Habr-Gama A, Sabbaga J, Gama-Rodrigues J, et al. Watch and wait approach following extended neoadjuvant chemoradiation for distal rectal cancer: are we getting closer to anal cancer management? *Dis Colon Rectum*. 2013;56(10):1109–17.
10. Maas M, Beets-Tan RG, Lambregts DM, et al. Wait-and-see policy for clinical complete responders after chemoradiation for rectal cancer. *J Clin Oncol*. 2011;29(35):4633–40.

11. Renehan AG, Malcomson L, Emsley R, et al. Watch-and-wait approach versus surgical resection after chemoradiotherapy for patients with rectal cancer (the OnCoRe project): a propensity-score matched cohort analysis. *Lancet Oncol.* 2016;17(2):174–83.
12. Smith JD, Ruby JA, Goodman KA, et al. Nonoperative management of rectal cancer with complete clinical response after neoadjuvant therapy. *Ann Surg.* 2012;256(6):965–72.
13. Spiegel DY, Boyer MJ, Hong JC, et al. Long-term clinical outcomes of nonoperative management with chemoradiotherapy for locally advanced rectal cancer in the veterans health administration. *Int J Radiat Oncol Biol Phys.* 2019;103(3):565–73.
14. Dossa F, Chesney TR, Acuna SA, Baxter NN. A watch-and-wait approach for locally advanced rectal cancer after a clinical complete response following neoadjuvant chemoradiation: a systematic review and meta-analysis. *Lancet Gastroenterol Hepatol.* 2017;2(7):501–13.
15. Dattani M, Heald RJ, Goussous G, et al. Oncological and survival outcomes in watch and wait patients with a clinical complete response after neoadjuvant chemoradiotherapy for rectal cancer: a systematic review and pooled analysis. *Ann Surg.* 2018;268(6):955–67.
16. van der Valk MJM, Hilling DE, Bastiaannet E, et al. Long-term outcomes of clinical complete responders after neoadjuvant treatment for rectal cancer in the International Watch & Wait Database (IWWD): an international multicentre registry study. *Lancet.* 2018;391(10139):2537–45.
17. Fernandez LM, São Julião GP, Figueiredo NL, et al. Conditional recurrence-free survival of clinical complete responders managed by watch and wait after neoadjuvant chemoradiotherapy for rectal cancer in the International Watch & Wait Database: a retrospective, international, multicentre registry study. *Lancet Oncol.* 2021;22(1):43–50.
18. Fernandez LM, São Julião GP, Renehan AG, et al. The risk of distant metastases in patients with clinical complete response managed by watch and wait after neoadjuvant therapy for rectal cancer: the influence of local regrowth in the international watch and wait database. *Dis Colon Rectum.* 2023;66(1):41–9.
19. Bahadoer RR, Peeters K, Beets GL, et al. Watch and wait after a clinical complete response in rectal cancer patients younger than 50 years. *Br J Surg.* 2021;109(1):114–20.
20. Zaborowski AM, Murphy B, Creavin B, et al. Clinicopathological features and oncological outcomes of patients with young-onset rectal cancer. *Br J Surg.* 2020;107(5):606–12.
21. Garcia-Aguilar J, Patil S, Gollub MJ, et al. Organ preservation in patients with rectal adenocarcinoma treated with total neoadjuvant therapy. *J Clin Oncol.* 2022;40(23):2546–56.
22. Conroy T, Bosset JF, Etienne PL, et al. Neoadjuvant chemotherapy with FOLFIRINOX and preoperative chemoradiotherapy for patients with locally advanced rectal cancer (UNICANCER-PRODIGE 23): a multicentre, randomised, open-label, phase 3 trial. *Lancet Oncol.* 2021;22(5):702–15.
23. Fokas E, Schlenska-Lange A, Polat B, et al. Chemoradiotherapy plus induction or consolidation chemotherapy as total neoadjuvant therapy for patients with locally advanced rectal cancer: long-term results of the CAO/ARO/AIO-12 randomized clinical trial. *JAMA Oncol.* 2022;8(1):e215445.
24. Cercek A, Lumish M, Sinopoli J, et al. PD-1 blockade in mismatch repair-deficient, locally advanced rectal cancer. *N Engl J Med.* 2022;386(25):2363–76.
25. Gani C, Gani N, Zschaeck S, et al. Organ preservation in rectal cancer: the patients' perspective. *Front Oncol.* 2019;9:318.

7

Patient setup, instrumentation, complications, and tips and tricks in transanal endoscopic surgery

Michael E. Kelly and Matthew R. Albert

Introduction

Traditionally, transanal surgery was limited to favourable low rectal (benign) lesions, as there were concerns over high rates of recurrence and compromised oncological outcomes.[1–5] However, with the development of transanal microsurgery (TEMS), which was first described in Germany in the 1980s, it has facilitated better accessibility for intraluminal resection of mid and upper rectal lesions.[6] Though originally designed for the removal of large polyps, it has evolved to include the excision of early rectal cancers.[7] Ultimately, the aim of local excision is to provide similar oncological and survival outcomes, while improving/maintaining the quality of life of the patient.

TEMS surgery marks the earliest reporting of natural office transluminal endoscopic surgery (NOTES). Since first being reported in the 1980s, its use has substantially increased across Europe, Australasia, and North America. However, the main limitations to widespread dissemination have been the acquisition of the specialized equipment (cost barriers) and the necessary specialist training.[8]

As a result, the development of transanal minimally invasive surgery (TAMIS) was pioneered in 2009 as an alternative to TEMS. It was designed to provide the surgeon with the advantage of TEMS, but offered a more flexible, simpler and cost-effective transanal platform.[9] TAMIS is performed via a single-access multichannel port, whereby laparoscopic instruments and endoscopic camera are inserted and the insufflator attached. The ergonomics are improved, there is better visualization (360 degrees) and similarities with single-port laparoscopic surgery reduce the learning curve issues. Its popularity has significantly increased in 10 years since being described, and it is now the leading transanal surgical platform.[8,10,11]

Patient selection, preparation, and standard practices

All patients being considered for transanal surgery should undergo a thorough history and clinical examination. Assessment of the patient's fitness and general wellbeing are important considerations. Routine investigations, including basic laboratory tests and carcinoembryonic antigen (CEA) levels, are important. Rectal examination is vital to note the location of the rectal lesion, its relationship with the sphincter complex and its characteristics (fixed, mobile, firmness, etc). Rigid sigmoidoscopy is also performed to assess the distance from the anal verge, position in relation to the rectal valves and luminal extent (percentage involvement). Finally, full colonoscopy is needed to out-rule synchronous lesions and facilitates biopsy of the lesion (if needed).

TEMS and TAMIS are suitable options for large polyps or early-stage rectal cancer (T1N0).[12] The use of transanal surgery in T2 lesions is controversial, due to risk of mesorectal nodal disease. Therefore prior to considering transanal surgery all patients must be accurately staged with endoscopic evaluation (with/without endorectal ultrasound) and cross-sectional imaging with computed tomography and magnetic resonance imaging (MRI) of the abdomen and pelvis. MRI is the most sensitive modality for assessing nodal involvement.[13]

In addition, it is vital to know the lesion size and location for planning purposes, and to plan patient positioning at the time of surgery. It also provides critical information in determining risk of peritoneal entry during dissection, which is also important to consider when consenting patients.[14] Patients are preoperatively assessed, anticoagulation is discontinued (bridging therapy commenced as needed), and patients are counselled regarding risks of surgery (explained next). Additionally, the possibility of histopathological upstaging of the tumour, requiring further radical surgery must be explained.

Mechanical bowel preparation, antimicrobial, and antithrombotic prophylaxis are routine practices. In some centres, bowel preparation with enemas is sufficient for low rectal lesions. Patients should be consented for laparoscopy/laparotomy with/without covering stoma in case of adverse event. The majority of patients have a general anaesthesia with endotracheal intubation to provide optimal paralysis.

For TEMS, as the tumour must be visible in the lower part of the rectoscope, patient positioning is essential (prone for anterior lesions, and lithotomy for posterior lesions). Alternatively, in TAMIS the majority of lesions can be excised in a lithotomy position.

Following antiseptic skin preparation and draping, the specific transanal platforms can be set up (discussed next). Rectal distension is facilitated via an insufflation system, and pneumorectum is maintained to facilitate dissection. There are two main options for insufflation; conventional insufflators, with a discontinuous flow (requiring the surgeon to open valve to evacuate the surgical plume), or continuous pressure systems that facilitate smoke evacuation and carbon dioxide recirculation throughout the procedure. More recently, an insufflation stabilization bag has been developed and used in conjunction with insufflators to minimize variations in pressure.[15,16]

Initially the operator marks out a 5–10 mm margin around the lesion and the dissection starts with a full-thickness proctotomy using monopolar cautery distal to the lesion. The use of an energy device is useful to maintain haemostasis but is an additional, often unnecessary expense. Care must be taken to avoid entering the abdominal cavity, for anterior lesions. Where possible, the excision defect is closed transversely to avoid rectal stenosis. Closure can be achieved in a continuous or interrupted fashion with absorbable sutures. The routine closure of all defects is debated, and there remains no international consensus. The majority of patients can be discharged the same day with a course of antimicrobial therapy (depending on local guidelines).[11,17,18]

Instrumentation techniques

Transanal endoscopic microsurgery (TEMS)

TEMS was developed by Buess and the Richard Wolf Medical Instruments Company in Germany in the 1980s.[6,7] Though originally developed for the removal of large rectal polyps it quickly expanded to include the excision of early-stage rectal neoplasms.

Using a rigid proctoscope platform (4 cm in diameter), it provides endoluminal insufflation to facilitate dissection anywhere in the rectum. A binocular optic is passed into the proctoscope to provide 3D views. Alternatively, a standard laparoscopic camera can be attached to a separate optic and connected to a video monitor. Instruments (5 mm) are then introduced through dedicated ports, which are similar to laparoscopic devices (graspers, scissors, needle holders, clip appliers, and cautery). TEMS uses a closed system with an airtight seal to ensure ease of dissection.

Patients are positioned specifically, in the prone position for anterior lesions and in lithotomy when the lesion is located posteriorly. The proctoscope is fixed in place by attaching it to a three-elbowed device (Martin Arm), which is then attached to the operating table. Prior to dissection, the margins are marked (1 cm) with cautery, and then lidocaine with adrenaline is instilled beneath the lesion to raise it. Using cautery, the lesion is then excised circumferentially in the full-thickness plane.

Transanal minimally invasive surgery (TAMIS)

For the majority of TAMIS cases, the lesion can be excised from the lithotomy position with the surgeon between the patient's legs. However, the prone position is utilized for some surgeons to facilitate resection of anterior tumours.

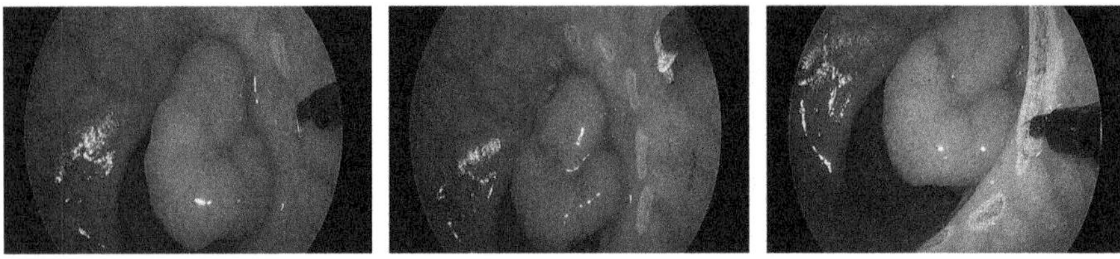

Fig. 7.1 Excision is typically performed with hook diathermy (monopolar) with a 5–10 mm margin.

Initially rectal examination is performed and the Lone Star Retractor System (Cooper Surgical, USA) is applied to expose the anal canal. The introduction of the TAMIS device is then placed. Total setup time is typically 3–5 minutes. The choice of the TAMIS platform is based on the surgeon's preference. GelPOINT (Applied Medical, USA) and SILS port (Medtronic, USA) are the two most commonly used devices. After deployment of the port, the pneumorectum is established with an initial pressure set at 15 mmHg. Increasing pressures up to 20 mm may be needed to maximize insufflation in the obese. The use of a 30 or 45 degree endoscope provides good views of the rectum, especially if the lesion transverses a rectal valve. Alternatively, some advocate the use of flexible endoscope and/or angulated instruments to reduce clashing of instruments.

To ensure an intact surgical specimen with clear margin is achieved, it is important to initially score the mucosa as a roadmap for excision. In the setting of larger lesions circumferential marking is not always possible, however, in the course of resection, the remaining areas should be marked as visualization permits. Excision is typically performed with hook diathermy (monopolar) with a 5–10 mm margin (Fig. 7.1). Bipolar devices are useful for control of bleeding vessels (but are associated with higher operative costs). In lesions that are concerning for neoplasm, a full-thickness excision with 10 mm margins is required. Dissection should be performed between the rectal wall and the surrounding mesorectal fat, controlling the perforating blood vessels. Handling of the polyp should be kept to a minimum to prevent fragmentation. For lesions that are clearly benign, a partial-thickness, or submucosal excision could be considered, using a submucosal lift with adrenaline-saline solution.

Rectal wall/mucosal defects are typically closed in a full-thickness manner with absorbable sutures. The use of V-Loc suture (Medtronic, USA) or laparoscopic knot pushers has made this process more efficient (Fig. 7.2).

Postoperative management

The majority of patients can be operated on an outpatient basis. However, in patients with advanced age, significant comorbidities or with increased risk of bleeding (on anticoagulant, underlying medical conditions, etc.), selective overnight

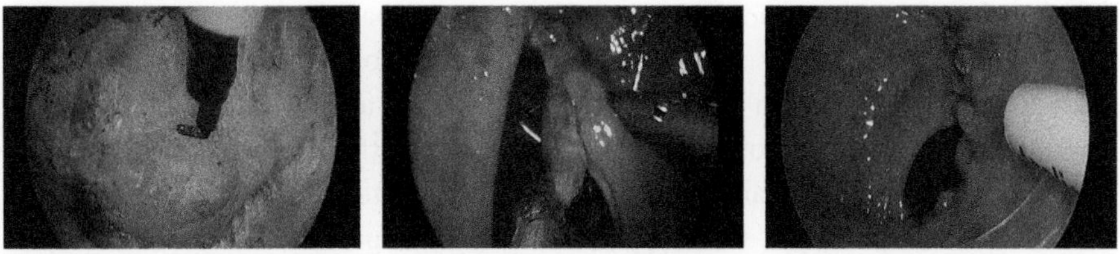

Fig. 7.2 Defect at the end of submucosal excision. Rectal wall defects are typically closed in a full-thickness manner with absorbable sutures.

admission should be considered. All patients must be counselled regarding early/late haemorrhage and rectal sepsis. It is often routine that patients are discharged on antimicrobials, for which the type and length should be dependent on local guidelines. Patients should be aware they will experience a change in bowel motion for several days post-procedure, but pain issues should be minimal, as these lesions are above the dentate line. Therefore, simple analgesia should suffice. If the abdominal cavity has be inadvertently entered, the patient is typically admitted for 24 hours of clinical observation.

Complications

Complications following TEMS or TAMIS are relatively low in incidence and severity when compared with radical surgery. The most common transient issues are urinary retention and faecal incontinence, especially following TEMS (0–11%).[10,19] The incontinence is likely due to continuous anal dilatation from the access channel and prolonged duration of surgery.[20] Karakayli *et al.* examined anorectal function following TAMIS surgery, noting no difference in anorectal manometry or Cleveland Clinic Incontinence Scores at six weeks.[21] A literature review by Palmieri et al., demonstrated good anorectal function and quality of life with both TEM and TAMIS, without postoperative sequelae at mid-term follow-up.[22]

Bleeding is another common complication following any transanal resection (0.7–9%). In most instances, it is self-limited. It can occur early or late, with late bleeds being associated with defect dehiscence. In most cases, supportive care is ample; alternatively, colonoscopy and coagulation treatment can be considered. Rarely, patients need to be brought back to the operative room for over-sewing of the bleeding vessel.[12,23]

Fever has been reported as a common event following transanal surgery. Theoretically, it is postulated that this is due to a transient bacteraemia and is self-limiting. If persistence of high temperatures or other signs of systematic inflammatory response are observed it mandates further investigation.

Peritoneal entry is potentially one of the more serious complications of transanal surgery (~4%).[24] The peritoneal reflection can vary considerably in both males and females; therefore, the operating surgeon must be prepared to encounter this challenge, especially in upper or mid-rectal anterior lesions. Historically, peritoneal entry required conversion to laparotomy, resection, and possible creation of a stoma. Nowadays, most would close the defect by full-thickness suture transanally. Alternatively, laparoscopy and defect closure, with leak test and/or possible covering stoma, is widely practised. One specific concern with peritoneal entry is the compromise to oncological safety, especially with early rectal cancers. There are concerns that this causes peritoneal seeding, with increased local recurrence.[25] However, multiple studies have not supported this belief.

Dehiscence of the wound defect closure site probably happens more often than reported. In most instances, it is self-limited with minor discharge.[26] Infection does not seem to be a common issue, as the majority of patients are discharged on antimicrobial therapy. Perez *et al.* reported suture line dehiscence rates of 61%, with only 43% of patients requiring admission for management.[27] However, suture line dehiscence after peritoneal entry does carry the potential of pelvic sepsis, and therefore is understandably feared. Reports of severe sepsis requiring laparotomy and faecal diversion have been reported, but with secure closure seldom occurring. Finally, other rare complications included rectovaginal fistulae (0.3–1.4%) that, in some instances, may require temporary faecal diversion. Though not reported, the risk of urethral injury is a potential concern with bulky anterior lesions.[12,28]

Tips and tricks

Early learning phase

In the early phase of learning TEMS or TAMIS, careful patient selection is key. Posterior, mid-rectal lesions that are less than 3 cm are ideal first cases. Ensuring good positioning with the patient in high lithotomy optimizes the ergonomics and ensures surgeon comfort. In addition, complete muscle paralysis with endotracheal intubation will provide for ideal insufflation and exposure. Pre-marking/scoring the mucosa before formal excision and starting from distal to proximal helps to ensure good dissection and maintains specimen orientation.

Insufflation

Adequate insufflation is a critical component of a successful procedure. Ideally, the surgeon wants a distended and tensed rectum for the duration of the dissection. Insufflation should be performed through the top port to avoid insufflating through pooled blood. Most procedures can be completed with the insufflator set to 15 mmHg pressure. However, in obese patients, higher flows may be required. Pressures as high as 25 mmHg can be achieved using bariatric insufflators, with no reports of barotrauma or other adverse events. The use of an insufflation stabilization bag can significantly improve the function of conventional insufflators.

Irrigation

Irrigation of the excision bed initially with copious amounts of water, and having the patients' blood pressure at their own normal baseline ensures complete hemostasis. Some also advocate irrigating the excision site with dilute betadine, as it has some antidotal tumoricidal and bactericidal effects.

Suturing the defect

This is often reported as being one of the most technically difficult aspects of the procedure due to limited working space. The use of a self-locking suture, which permits avoidance of knot tying (V-Lok suture; Medtronic, USA), is run in a continuous fashion and expedites closure.

Conclusion

Historically, oncological outcomes from local excision for the treatment of early rectal cancer or large polyps have been disappointing. However, with improved surgical technology and platforms, and in appropriately selected patients, local excision via the transanal approach offers acceptable oncological resection with less morbidity.

References

1. Palmer G, Martling A, Cedermark B, Holm T. A population based study on the management and outcomes in patients with locally advanced rectal cancer. *Ann Surg Oncol.* 2007;14:447–54.
2. Morino M, Risio M, Bach S, Beets-Tan R, et al. Early rectal cancer: the European Association for Endoscopic Surgery (EAES) clinical consensus conference. *Surg Endosc.* 2015;29(4):755–73.
3. Garcia-Florez LJ, Otero-Diez JL. Local excision by transanal endoscopic surgery. *World J Gastrolenterol.* 2015;21(31):9286–96.
4. Lee L, Burke JP, deBeche-Adams T, et al. Transanal minimally invasive surgery for local excision of benign and malignant rectal neoplasia: outcomes from 200 consecutive cases with midterm follow up. *Ann Surg.* 2018;267(5):910–16.
5. Westrich G, Venturero M, Schtrechman G, et al. Transanal minimally invasive surgery for benign and malignant rectal lesions: operative and oncological outcomes of a single center experience. *J Laproendosc Adv Surg Tech.* 2019;29(9):1122–7.

6. Buess G, Theiss R, Hutterer F, et al. Transanal endoscopic surgery of the rectum—testing a new method in animal experiments. *Leber Magen Darm*. 1983;13(2):73–7.
7. Buess G, Mentges B, Manncke K, et al. Technique and results of transanal endoscopic microsurgery in early rectal cancer. *Am J Surg*. 1992;163:63–9; discussion 69–70.
8. Althumairi AA, Gearhart SL. Local excision for early rectal cancer: transanal endoscopic microsurgery and beyond. *J Gastrointest Oncol*. 2015;6(3):296–306.
9. Atallah S, Albert M, Larach S. Transanal minimally invasive surgery: a giant leap forward. *Surg Endosc*. 2010;24(9):2200–5.
10. Martin-Perez B, Andrade-Ribeiro GD, Hunter L, et al. A systematic review of transanal minimally invasive surgery (TAMIS) from 2010 to 2013. *Tech Coloproctol*. 2014;18:775–88.
11. Albert MR, Atallah SB, deBeche-Adams TC, Izfar S, Larach SW. Transanal minimally invasive surgery (TAMIS) for local excision of benign neoplasms and early-stage rectal cancer: efficacy and outcomes in the first 50 patients. *Dis Colon Rectum*. 2013;56(3):301–7.
12. Rai V, Mishra N. Transanal approach to rectal polyps and cancer. *Clin Colon Rectal Surg*. 2016; 29(1):65–70.
13. Patel RK, Sayers AE, Kumar P, Khulusi S, Razack A, Hunter IA. The role of endorectal ultrasound and magnetic resonance imaging in the management of early rectal lesions in a tertiary center. *Clin Colorectal Cancer*. 2014;13(4):245–50.
14. Brown G. Thin section MRI in multidisciplinary pre-operative decision making for patients with rectal cancer. *Br J Radiol*. 2005;78:S117–27.
15. Zoller S, Joos A, Dinter D, et al. Retrorectal tumors: excision by transanal endoscopic microsurgery. *Rev Esp Enferm Dig*. 2007;99:547–50.
16. Barendse RM, Dijkgraaf MG, Rolf UR, et al. Colorectal surgeons' learning curve of transanal endoscopic microsurgery. *Surg Endosc*. 2013;27:3591–602.
17. Lee L, Kelly J, Nassif GJ, et al. Establishing the learning curve of transanal minimally invasive surgery for local excision of rectal neoplasms. *Surg Endosc*. 2018;32(3):1368–76.
18. Lee L, Edwards K, Hunter IA, et al. Quality of local excision for rectal neoplasms using transanal endoscopic microsurgery versus transanal minimally invasive surgery: a multi-institutional matched analysis. *Dis Colon Rectum*. 2017;60(9):928–35.
19. Ondhia M, Tamvakeras P, O'Toole P, et al. Transanal endoscopic microsurgery for rectal lesions in a specialist regional early rectal cancer centre: the Mersey experience. *Colorectal Dis*. 2019;21(10):1164–74.
20. Jakubauskas M, Jotautas V, Poskus E, et al. Fecal incontinence after transanal endoscopic microsurgery. *Int J Colorectal Dis*. 2018;33(4):467–72.
21. Karakayali FY, Tezcaner T, Moray G. Anorectal function and outcomes after transanal minimally invasive surgery for rectal tumors. *J Minim Access Surg*. 2015;11(4):257–62.
22. Palmieri L, Corallino D, Manni R, Meoli F, Paganini AM. Quality of life and anorectal function after transanal surgery for rectal cancer. A literature review. *Ann Ital Chir*. 2019;90:138–44.
23. Dias AR, Nahas CSR, Marques CFS, Nahas SC, Cecconello I. Transanal endoscopic microsurgery: indications, results and controversies. *Tech Coloproctol*. 2009;13(2):105–11.
24. Heidary B, Phang T P, Raval M J, Brown C J. Transanal endoscopic microsurgery: a review. *Can J Surg*. 2014;57(2):127–38.
25. Whitehouse PA, Tilney HS, Armitage JN, et al. Transanal endoscopic microsurgery: risk factors for local recurrence of benign rectal adenomas. *Colorectal Dis*. 2006;8:795–9.
26. Menahem B, Alves A, Morello R, Lubrano J. Should the rectal defect be closed following transanal local excision of rectal tumors? A systematic review and meta-analysis. *Tech Coloproctol*. 2017;21(12):929–36.

27. Perez RO, Habr-Gama A, São Julião GP, et al. Transanal endoscopic microsurgery for residual rectal cancer after neoadjuvant chemoradiation therapy is associated with significant immediate pain and hospital readmission rates. *Dis Colon Rectum*. 2011;54(5):545–51.
28. Clancy C, Burke JP, Albert MR, O'Connell PR, Winter DC. Transanal endoscopic microsurgery versus standard transanal excision for the removal of rectal neoplasms: a systematic review and meta-analysis. *Dis Colon Rectum*. 2015;58(2):254–61.

8

Local excision for early rectal cancers

James Glasbey, Roel Hompes, and Simon Bach

Introduction

Total mesorectal excision (TME) surgery is considered the gold standard for the management of rectal cancer, including most early-stage rectal cancer. In the UK, 27% of TME operations are performed for non-irradiated T1 and T2 rectal tumours.[1] While TME surgery provides effective local tumour control, up to 40% of patients experience serious complications, with relatively high rates of acute and late patient-reported side effects that reduce overall quality of life, social function, and body image while increasing embarrassment about bowel function.[2,3] Introduction of population bowel screening, increased bowel cancer awareness, and expedient investigation of new bowel symptoms all promote the detection of rectal cancer at an early stage. At diagnosis, screened patients with early rectal cancer may be asymptomatic, relatively young, and in good health. The risks of morbidity and functional impairment associated with TME surgery may feel unacceptably high to these individuals. Meanwhile, in older patients the presence of frailty or multiple morbidity heightens the risks associated with radical surgical treatment.[4] Organ preservation aims to avoid radical surgery thereby reducing treatment-related morbidity to improve patients' quality of life. An organ-preserving approach may involve local transanal surgery, radiotherapy or chemotherapy/immunotherapy, either individually or in combination.[5] While clinicians and patients recognize the potential benefits of an organ preservation approach for treatment of early rectal cancer, there remain barriers to widespread adoption. For instance, in early rectal cancer the primary tumour may appear amenable to transanal local excision, however, multiple case series report poor long-term oncological results with local recurrence rates ranging from 5% to 28% for T1 lesions, and 11% to 45% for T2 lesions.[6,7] In addition, trials of radiotherapy followed by local excision consistently identify toxicity arising from multiple treatments as problematic, particularly for those patients who do not achieve organ preservation, although recent inroads have been made.[2,8] In this chapter, we will describe the platforms for local excision of early rectal cancers, consider patient selection and discuss the clinical and pathological outcomes of local excision without neoadjuvant therapy.

Transanal endoscopic surgery

Transanal endoscopic microsurgery (TEM) was developed by Buess in the 1980s to provide an optimized endoluminal operating platform for the removal of benign rectal adenomas.[9] The TEM equipment incorporates an operating proctoscope, endoscopic 3D binocular viewer, and modified laparoscopic instruments. The proctoscope is designed to keep an airtight seal around the anal verge, and the operating field is pressure-regulated to minimize movement of the operative field. The faceplate of the proctoscope admits the endoscopic camera, a suction device, and two instruments. These instruments are either straight, for access to the lateral aspects of the operative field or angulated near their tip to improve range of motion, which is useful for access to the lower area. The original TEM platform has spawned many imitators such as transanal minimally invasive surgery (TAMIS) and transanal endoscopic operation (TEO), reflecting the increasing popularity of transanal techniques and an expanding range of indications.[10–13] Collectively these are often referred to as transanal endoscopic surgery (TES). Platforms generally dispense with the binocular view and pressure-regulated operating field, instead utilizing conventional laparoscopic equipment to somewhat reduce costs. Proctorship in TES with an experienced trainer is essential, with a comparable learning curve to that seen for laparoscopic colorectal resection.[14,15] However, one of the great strengths of the TES platform is that novices can learn the various techniques by enrolling in courses that provide very realistic simulation. Optimized techniques of local transanal excision via TES reduce rates of margin positivity, fragmented specimens, and local recurrence compared to older styles of per anal excision using retractors and diathermy.[16,17]

Identification and assessment of early-stage rectal cancer

Presentation of early-stage rectal cancer follows two common scenarios. Firstly, a polyp has already been locally removed, and histopathology identifies a focus of malignancy. The multidisciplinary team (MDT) must consider how best to advise the patient, and local transanal excision of the polyp base may be considered to evaluate completeness of excision. If re-excision reveals no further tumour or minimal residual disease, then organ preservation may be considered. Secondly, the patient is referred to the MDT with a significant rectal polyp. There may be clinical concerns that this polyp is malignant, or biopsies reveal either intramucosal high-grade dysplasia or definite malignant invasion of the submucosa. Establishing the correct diagnosis at the outset is important as this enables patients to consider a full range of therapeutic options. Where malignancy is clinically suspected or biopsies report diffuse high-grade dysplastic changes, then specialist evaluation should be sought with a low threshold for repeat examination and further biopsy by an experienced practitioner. Low rectal tumours are particularly prone to superficial endoscopic biopsy that fails to demonstrate tumour invasion due to a tangential angle of approach created when the rectum is inflated by a scope situated only a short distance away in the anal canal. Inverting the scope via the J manoeuvre can help to obtain deeper samples.

Irrespective of the clinical scenario, all patients who present with significant rectal lesions should undergo standard TNM staging and visualization of the whole colon, looking for synchronous bowel pathology. High-quality staging investigations not only serve to identify occasional cases of advanced disease or a second significant pathology but provide a valuable baseline reference for patients who enter a programme of close observation following organ preservation. Staging investigations preformed after polypectomy can reveal 'reactive' lymphadenopathy, however such findings resolve as the mucosal wound heals. Features of nodal irregularity, mixed signal intensity or loss of chemical shift artefact on MRI are all highly suggestive of nodal involvement and would prompt serious consideration of a radical surgical approach. However, the overall performance of MRI in staging early rectal cancer is disappointing, both with respect to tumour and nodal staging.[18] Dutch population-based analysis highlights overstaging of pT1 tumours in 54.7% of cases using MRI alone and 31% if MRI is combined with endorectal ultrasound, limiting the application of local excision for pT1 tumours.[18] Conversely, staging often also fails to appreciate features considered high risk for relapse following local excision. Studies such as TESAR are exploring if it is possible to compensate for inaccurate staging following local excision through application of chemoradiotherapy versus immediately converting to TME.[19]

Full-thickness transanal endoscopic surgery for rectal cancer

Where a rectal polyp is known to be malignant and TES intended as curative then resection should be full thickness, including the muscularis propria. Incorporating a mucosal margin of 10 mm around the tumour allows grasping and manipulation without touching or macerating the tumour. After full-thickness excision, the defect should be closed to heal by primary intention. Closure may be more difficult for tumours situated near the anal verge. The highest lesions that are amenable to endoscopic excision using this technique are typically around 25 cm from the anal verge.[20] One limitation is the ability to negotiate the TES equipment past the bony sacrum.

The great advantage of TES is that it consistently yields an en bloc local tumour specimen for histopathological evaluation. The tumour is definitively characterized as benign or malignant by the presence of submucosal invasion. Tumour diameter, depth of invasion, grade, and resection margin status are recorded. T1 tumours are subclassified according to progression through the submucosa as sm1, 2, or 3. The presence of intramural lymphatic or vascular invasion is recorded. This critical information is used to stratify an individual's risk of local relapse.[6,7] In contrast, piecemeal endoscopic mucosal resection (EMR) does not provide high-quality pathology

Table 8.1 Local recurrence rates at three years following transanal endoscopic surgery for early-stage rectal cancer. Reproduced with permission of *BJS*[6]

		Maximum tumour diameter (cm)					
Depth of Invasion	LY V	≤1	1.1–2	2.1–3	3.1–4	4.1–5	5.1+
pT1 sm1	–	3.0	3.6	4.4	5.4	6.6	8.1
	+	5.2	6.4	7.7	9.4	11.4	13.7
pT1 sm2 pT1 sm3	–	10.5	12.7	15.3	18.5	22.1	26.4
	+	17.8	21.4	25.5	30.3	35.7	41.8
pT2	–	9.8	11.9	14.3	17.3	20.7	24.7
	+	16.7	20.0	23.9	28.5	33.7	39.5

specimens, so staging information is lost, potentially predisposing to overtreatment with radical surgery.

Full-thickness TEM without neoadjuvant therapy can only really be considered as a curative treatment for a very selected group of low-risk pT1 cancer (Table 8.1).[6,21] These are generally smaller lesions, less than 3 cm in maximum diameter, without evidence of adverse features that include high-grade, intramural lymphatic invasion or intramural vascular invasion. Local relapse rates at three years following full-thickness TEM for sm1 early rectal cancer without high-risk features are in the order of 5%.[6] Patients have excellent quality of life benefits, with low risk of relapse.[22] However, it is also clear that a significant proportion of early tumours exhibit less favourable histopathological features (e.g. Kikuchi *sm2* or *sm3* disease, or with (lympho)vascular invasion) and consequently relapse more frequently.[6,7] Here, transanal surgery clearly represents a compromise.[6,23] Currently, the accuracy and precision of diagnostic testing are insufficient to reliably guide treatment, and this limits the usefulness of local excision in early rectal cancer.[18] The true nature of a tumour may only become apparent once it is removed, prompting conversion to total mesorectal excision (TME) or a range of somewhat experimental therapies, including contact and external beam chemoradiotherapy.[19] It is therefore of paramount importance that the implications of conversion to TME are appreciated and discussed upfront, prior to embarking upon any treatment. Completion (secondary) TME increases the risk of stoma and may yield a perforated specimen compared to primary TME.[24] Full-thickness TES will encroach upon the circumferential resection margin anteriorly; in the event of local recurrence, this strategy could result in pelvic exenteration. Exposing the pelvic floor when performing TES low in the rectum may mean that subsequent conversion to TME is via extralevator abdominoperineal excision.

The role of partial thickness transanal endoscopic surgery

TES platforms such as TEM allow the operator to perform a range of different operations including mucosectomy, submucosal incision, dissection between the layers of the muscularis propria, or beyond into mesorectal fat.[12] While full-thickness excision facilitates clear margins, particularly in cases that are understaged preoperatively, this strategy risks jeopardizing the integrity of the circumferential resection both anteriorly and low in the rectum. Partial thickness excision of the submucosa, leaving the muscularis propria intact, can be a useful strategy in selected cases where there is diagnostic doubt or an awkward tumour location. Tumours may be excised *en bloc*, the presence of a malignant component is established, while also minimizing the risks associated with subsequent conversion to TME.

Partial thickness excision via endoscopic submucosal dissection (ESD) is a minimally invasive en bloc resection technique that provides an alternative to TES. ESD is gaining popularity for the treatment of superficial colorectal neoplasms. TRIASSiC is an ongoing trial comparing endoscopic submucosal dissection (ESD) and transanal minimal invasive surgery (TAMIS) for resection of non-pedunculated rectal lesions, with results expected within the next three years, which will add clarity to the surgeons' choice of procedural selection.[25]

Intraperitoneal dissection

Peritoneal breach during TES is generally considered safe, both in terms of oncological outcomes and adverse events.[26–29] Defects are amenable to sutured repair via TES or alternatively using laparoscopic instruments if access from below is inadequate. It may be advisable to observe patients overnight, and evaluation with a water-soluble contrast enema prior to discharge can provide additional reassurance.

Surveillance following TES

Surveillance schedules evolved somewhat empirically and have been driven by a desire not to miss treatable regrowths. A popular approach is to evaluate the patient every three months during the first two years when the risk of relapse is greatest (Fig. 8.1). Subsequently, six-monthly intervals are advised for five years. Local evaluation takes the form of direct visualization of the bowel wall and cross-sectional imaging of the mesorectum and pelvis. We favour flexible endoscopy with a phosphate enema bowel preparation and high-quality MRI. It is important to remember that 1520% of cases will relapse with metastatic disease. We therefore advise CT thorax, abdomen and pelvis annually up to three years, in line with our other colorectal cancer patients.

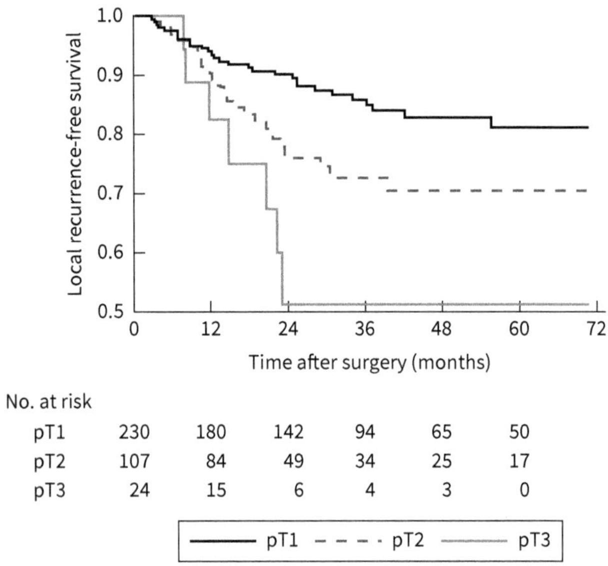

Fig. 8.1 Risk of local relapse over time according to pT stage.
Reproduced with permission of *BJS*.[6]

Summary and future perspectives

Invention of the TEM platform enabled us to reliably deliver minimally invasive treatment for large benign rectal polyps. The hope that early cancers might also be amenable to local excision with good results sadly did not materialize, largely because of current limitations in preoperative staging. While early rectal cancer can be resected using TES with reduced morbidity and better functional outcomes compared to TME, local cancer recurrence is problematic, and it is suggested that long-term survival with TES is worse than TME.[7] To some extent, worse long-term outcomes may reflect the fact that TES may be offered to individuals considered high risk for TME as a compromise solution. However, it is impossible to overlook the fact that TES frequently yields specimens where the predicted rate of local recurrence may be between 20–30%. Why do so many patients relapse locally? Technical factors include the plane of excision and tumour cell implantation during TES. Even in expert hands, R1 resection has been observed in 10% of pT1 and 20% of pT2 cases.[6] Biological factors include discontinuous tumour spread via blood vessels and lymphatics. Current guidelines recommend that TEMS alone without neoadjuvant therapy should be reserved for very early rectal cancers (pT1) with favourable clinical and histopathological characteristics (for example, sm1cN0).[30,31] This is however a problematic strategy as histopathological factors are only recognized in retrospect. These limitations prompted a series of studies to evaluate neoadjuvant therapy prior to TES to combat technical and biological treatment failure. Studies included TREC, CARTS, ACOSOG Z6041, and GRECCAR-2.[2,32–34] The field of organ preservation continues to evolve through trials such as STAR-TREC with introduction of smaller, mesorectal radiation fields and selective TES following complete response.[8,35]

References

1. ACPGBI. National bowel cancer audit. 2021. https://www.nboca.org.uk/reports/annual-report-2021/.
2. Bach SP, Gilbert A, Brock K, et al. Radical surgery versus organ preservation via short-course radiotherapy followed by transanal endoscopic microsurgery for early-stage rectal cancer (TREC): a randomised, open-label feasibility study. *Lancet Gastroenterol Hepatol.* 2021;6(2):92–105.
3. Bolton WS, Chapman SJ, Corrigan N, et al. The incidence of low anterior resection syndrome as assessed in an international randomized controlled trial (MRC/NIHR ROLARR). *Ann Surg.* 2021;274(6):e1223–e9.
4. Rutten HJT, den Dulk M, Lemmens VEPP, van de Velde CJH, Marijnen CAM. Controversies of total mesorectal excision for rectal cancer in elderly patients. *Lancet Oncol.* 2008;9(5):494–501.
5. Fleming C, Vendrely V, Rullier E, Denost Q. Organ preservation in rectal cancer: review of contemporary management. *Br J Surg.* 2022;109(8):695–703.
6. Bach SP, Hill J, Monson JR, et al. A predictive model for local recurrence after transanal endoscopic microsurgery for rectal cancer. *Br J Surg.* 2009;96(3):280–90.
7. Halverson AL, Morris AM, Cleary RK, Chang GJ. For patients with early rectal cancer, does local excision have an impact on recurrence, survival, and quality of life relative to radical resection? *Ann Surg Oncol.* 2019;26(8):2497–506.
8. Bach SP, Wilt JHWd, Peters F, et al. STAR-TREC phase II: Can we save the rectum by watchful waiting or transanal surgery following (chemo)radiotherapy versus total mesorectal excision for early rectal cancer? *J Clin Oncol.* 2022;40(16_suppl):3502.
9. Bretagnol F, Merrie A, George B, Warren BF, Mortensen NJ. Local excision of rectal tumours by transanal endoscopic microsurgery. *Br J Surg.* 2007;94(5):627–33.
10. Atallah S, Albert M, Larach S. Transanal minimally invasive surgery: a giant leap forward. *Surg Endosc.* 2010;24(9):2200–5.
11. D'Hondt M, Yoshihara E, Dedrye L, Vindevoghel K, Nuytens F, Pottel H. Transanal endoscopic operation for benign rectal lesions and T1 carcinoma. *JSLS.* 2017;21(1):e2016.00093.
12. Smart CJ, Cunningham C, Bach SP. Transanal endoscopic microsurgery. *Best Pract Res Clin Gastroenterol.* 2014;28(1):143–57.
13. Baatrup G, Breum B, Qvist N, et al. Transanal endoscopic microsurgery in 143 consecutive patients with rectal adenocarcinoma: results from a Danish multicenter study. *Colorectal Dis.* 2009;11(3):270–5.
14. Koebrugge B, Bosscha K, Ernst MF. Transanal endoscopic microsurgery for local excision of rectal lesions: is there a learning curve? *Dig Surg.* 2009;26(5):372–7.
15. Barendse RM, Dijkgraaf MG, Rolf UR, et al. Colorectal surgeons' learning curve of transanal endoscopic microsurgery. *Surg Endosc.* 2013;27(10):3591–602.
16. De Graaf EJ, Doornebosch PG, Tollenaar RA, et al. Transanal endoscopic microsurgery versus total mesorectal excision of T1 rectal adenocarcinomas with curative intention. *Eur J Surg Oncol.* 2009;35(12):1280–5.

17. Clancy C, Burke JP, Albert MR, O'Connell PR, Winter DC. Transanal endoscopic microsurgery versus standard transanal excision for the removal of rectal neoplasms: a systematic review and meta-analysis. *Dis Colon Rectum.* 2015;58(2):254–61.
18. Detering R, van Oostendorp SE, Meyer VM, et al. MRI cT1–2 rectal cancer staging accuracy: a population-based study. *Br J Surg.* 2020;107(10):1372–82.
19. Borstlap WA, Tanis PJ, Koedam TW, et al. A multi-centred randomised trial of radical surgery versus adjuvant chemoradiotherapy after local excision for early rectal cancer. *BMC Cancer.* 2016;16:513.
20. Papagrigoriadis S. Transanal endoscopic micro-surgery (TEMS) for the management of large or sessile rectal adenomas: a review of the technique and indications. *Int Semin Surg Oncol.* 2006;3:13.
21. Morino M, Risio M, Bach S, et al. Early rectal cancer: the European Association for Endoscopic Surgery (EAES) clinical consensus conference. *Surg Endosc.* 2015;29(4):755–73.
22. Ptok H, Marusch F, Meyer F, et al. Oncological outcome of local vs radical resection of low-risk pT1 rectal cancer. *Arch Surg.* 2007;142(7):649–55; discussion 56.
23. Suppiah A, Maslekar S, Alabi A, Hartley JE, Monson JR. Transanal endoscopic microsurgery in early rectal cancer: time for a trial? *Colorectal Dis.* 2008;10(4):314–27; discussion 27–9.
24. Eid Y, Alves A, Lubrano J, Menahem B. Does previous transanal excision for early rectal cancer impair surgical outcomes and pathologic findings of completion total mesorectal excision? Results of a systematic review of the literature. *J Visc Surg.* 2018;155(6):445–52.
25. Dekkers N, Boonstra JJ, Moons LMG, et al. Transanal minimally invasive surgery (TAMIS) versus endoscopic submucosal dissection (ESD) for resection of non-pedunculated rectal lesions (TRIASSIC study): study protocol of a European multicenter randomised controlled trial. *BMC Gastroenterol.* 2020;20(1):225.
26. Mege D, Petrucciani N, Maggiori L, Panis Y. Peritoneal perforation is less a complication than an expected event during transanal endoscopic microsurgery: experience from 194 consecutive cases. *Tech Coloproctol.* 2017;21(9):729–36.
27. Morino M, Allaix ME, Famiglietti F, Caldart M, Arezzo A. Does peritoneal perforation affect short- and long-term outcomes after transanal endoscopic microsurgery? *Surg Endosc.* 2013;27(1):181–8.
28. Baatrup G, Borschitz T, Cunningham C, Qvist N. Perforation into the peritoneal cavity during transanal endoscopic microsurgery for rectal cancer is not associated with major complications or oncological compromise. *Surg Endosc.* 2009;23(12):2680–3.
29. Gavagan JA, Whiteford MH, Swanstrom LL. Full-thickness intraperitoneal excision by transanal endoscopic microsurgery does not increase short-term complications. *Am J Surg.* 2004;187(5):630–4.
30. Morino M, Risio M, Bach S, et al. Early rectal cancer: the European Association for Endoscopic Surgery (EAES) clinical consensus conference. *Surg Endosc.* 2015;29(4):755–73.
31. Borstlap WAA, van Oostendorp SE, Klaver CEL, et al. Organ preservation in rectal cancer: a synopsis of current guidelines. *Colorectal Dis.* 2017. doi: 10.1111/codi.13960.
32. Verseveld M, de Graaf EJ, Verhoef C, et al. Chemoradiation therapy for rectal cancer in the distal rectum followed by organ-sparing transanal endoscopic microsurgery (CARTS study). *Br J Surg.* 2015;102(7):853–60.
33. Rullier E, Rouanet P, Tuech JJ, et al. Organ preservation for rectal cancer (GRECCAR 2): a prospective, randomised, open-label, multicentre, phase 3 trial. *Lancet.* 2017;390(10093):469–79.

34. Garcia-Aguilar J, Renfro LA, Chow OS, et al. Organ preservation for clinical t2n0 distal rectal cancer using neoadjuvant chemoradiotherapy and local excision: results of a multicenter phase 2 study. *Lancet Oncol.* 2015;16(15):1537–46.
35. Bach SP, Collaborative S-T. Can we Save the rectum by watchful waiting or TransAnal surgery following (chemo)Radiotherapy versus Total mesorectal excision for early REctal Cancer (STAR-TREC)? Protocol for the international, multicentre, rolling phase II/III partially randomized patient preference trial evaluating long-course concurrent chemoradiotherapy versus short-course radiotherapy organ preservation approaches. *Colorectal Dis.* 2022;24(5):639–51.

9
Local excision for locally advanced rectal cancer post neoadjuvant therapy

Tijmen Koëter, Rutger C.H. Stijns, and J.H.W. (Hans) de Wilt

Local excision following radiotherapy

When local excision after neoadjuvant radiotherapy as an organ-preserving treatment is pursued, generally two radiotherapy regimens are administered. Short-course radiotherapy, consisting of five fractions of 5 Gy in one week (5×5 Gy) versus long-course radiotherapy (i.e. five fractions of 1.8–2 Gy per week during 5–6 weeks) are both previously described as neoadjuvant treatment (Table 9.1).[1] Short-course neoadjuvant radiotherapy has shown to improve local recurrence rates when combined with TME surgery.[2] The Stockholm 3 trial aimed to study recurrence rates in patients between three different radiotherapy regimens.[3] One arm consisted of patients treated with short-course radiotherapy and a long interval to surgery (4–8 weeks), resulting in a ypT0 (pCR) rate of 11.8%. As such, short-course radiotherapy with a delayed assessment of tumour downstaging can be a treatment option for selected patients and especially for those who are unfit to undergo chemotherapy. Not only patients with a complete response, but also patients with a near-complete response (ypT1N0) could potentially be treated with local excision. In a study from the Dutch cancer registry, 17.5% of patients had a good pathological response (ypT0-1N0) after 5×5Gy radiotherapy and delayed TME surgery.[4] These patients were potential candidates for organ preservation when local excision was performed instead of radical surgery. Results from the Stockholm 3 trial showed that 6% of patients after short-course radiotherapy develop grade 3–4 radiation-induced toxicity requiring admittance during the resting period to surgery. Postoperative complication rate was significantly lower in the deferred surgery arm compared to the immediate surgery arm. Although there was no direct comparison with patients who underwent chemoradiation, these toxicity profiles seem to be rather mild. Little is known of the effect of short-course radiotherapy on clinical tumour response rates when evaluating for an organ-preserving intention. One study described a cohort of 62 patients treated with neoadjuvant short-course radiotherapy and a delayed local excision after 10–12 weeks.[5] Included patients were mostly frail and unfit for TME surgery, staged with cT1–2N0 tumours. Histopathological T stage in the resected specimens was ypT0 (pCR) for 20 patients (32%) (Table 9.1).

Table 9.1 Outcomes of local excision after neo-adjuvant treatment in rectal cancer

Study	No. of patients	Primary TN stage	Intervention	Follow-up	LR-free	DFS	DSS	OS	Organ preserved
Radiotherapy alone									
Lezoche et al., 2005	100	cT2N0	RT 50.4 Gy + TEM	90	95	NM	89	72	97
Smart et al., 2016	62	cT1-2N0	RT 25 Gy + TEM	24	89	77	NM	84	95
Bach et al., 2021	27	cT1-2N0	RT 25Gy + TEM	36	91	76	NM	86	70
Chemoradiotherapy									
Lezoche, 2008	35	cT2N0	RT 50.4 Gy + 5-FU + TEM	84	94	94	NM	97	94
Pucciarelli, 2013	63	cT2-3N0	RT 50.4 Gy + 5-FU + TEM	36	97	91	NM	92	82
Perez et al., 2013	27	cT2-4N0-2	RT 50.4-54 Gy + 5-FU + TEM	15	78	68	89	96	87
Perez, 2014	22	cT2N0	RT 50.4 Gy + 5-FU + TEM	22	83	NM	NM	NM	73
Garcia-Aguilar, 2015	79	cT2N0	RT 54 Gy + CAPOX + TEM	60	90	80	NM	91	91
Creavin et al., 2017	35	cT3-4N0-2	RT 50–54 Gy + 5-FU + TEM/TAMIS	29	91.4	80	NM	94.3	89
Rullier, 2017	71	cT2-3N0-1	RT 50 Gy + CAPOX + LE	36	95	78	NM	92	NM
Stijns, 2019	55	cT1-3N0-1	RT 50–50.4 Gy + CPC + TEM	53	91	81.6	NM	82.8	64
Cerra-Aracil, 2023	86	cT2-3abN0	RT 45 +5.4 Gy + 5-FU + TEM	1	NM	NM	NM	NM	83

RT, radiotherapy; Gy, gray; 5-FU, fluorouracil-based chemotherapy; CAPOX, capecitabin and oxaliplatin; CPC, capecitabin; UFT, tegafur-uracil; TEM, transanal endoscopic microsurgery; TAMIS, transanal minimally invasive surgery; LE, local excision; LR-free, local-recurrence-free; DFS, disease-free-survival; DSS, disease-specific survival; OS, overall survival; NM, not mentioned.

Lezoche et al. studied the effect of high-dose radiation therapy combined with local excision in patients with T2-3N0 distal rectal cancer, aiming to evaluate this treatment as a valid alternative to TME surgery.[1] A total of 100 patients (54 cT2 and 46 cT3) were enrolled and underwent high-dose radiotherapy (50.4 Gy, 28 fractions over five weeks) followed by local excision. After long-term follow-up (90 months), the cancer-specific survival rate was 89% and they reported an organ preservation rate of 97%. Regarding acute toxicity, skin erythema (66%) and diarrhoea (22%) were reported during the long-term radiotherapy course. Late toxicity after radiotherapy was not described in this study.

The TREC-collaborators recruited 55 patients, diagnosed with a cT1-2N0M0 rectal tumour with a maximum diameter of 30 mm, and randomized these patients to undergo organ preservation with short-course radiotherapy followed by local excision after 8–10 weeks versus total mesorectal excision (TME). At three-year follow-up, overall survival was 86% in the organ preservation group versus 100% in the radical surgery group ($p = 0.24$). Patients assigned to organ preservation showed improvements in patient-reported bowel toxicities and quality of life and function scores in multiple items compared to those assigned to total mesorectal excision.[6,7]

Local excision following chemoradiotherapy

Habr-Gama et al. were the first to describe a cCR of 26.8% in patients diagnosed with more advanced (T1>) rectal cancer treated with chemoradiotherapy (CRT).[8] Following this publication, several trials were conducted in which patients with intermediate-risk (T2-3N0-1) rectal cancers were treated with neoadjuvant (C)RT followed by local excision.[9–12] In these trials, patients with a significant response on MRI and/or endoscopy were selected for treatment with local excision or otherwise underwent standard TME surgery. Promising DFS and OS rates were achieved with high rates (64–97%) of successful organ preserving. It seems that local excision after CRT may be an oncologically safe equivalent to TME in selected patients with rectal cancer. Results from a meta-analysis of local excision after neoadjuvant treatment versus TME surgery showed that local recurrences rates were not significantly greater (10.1% local excision vs. 8% TME), and no difference in overall or disease-free survival (13). More recently, the TAUTEM study was published and reported the short-term outcomes of a randomized controlled trial comparing organ preservation using chemoradiotherapy followed by local excision versus standard of care TME surgery for patients with cT2-3abN0 rectal cancer. A total of 173 patients were included during an 11-year inclusion period. The short-term results showed an encouraging organ preservation rate of almost 83% in the organ preservation group. Long-term outcomes regarding overall survival as well as quality of life are to be awaited.[14]

Patients with locally advanced tumours (endangered mesorectal fascia or extensive lymph node involvement) are also eligible for organ-preserving treatment.

Pathological complete response following CRT in locally advanced rectal cancer (LARC) vary between 10 and 20% according to the literature.[15] Although numbers are still small, results suggests that local excision seems feasible in patient with LARC after CRT. Creavin et al. described 35 patients with LARC who underwent organ-preserving treatment after an objective endoluminal response to CRT, with a similar disease-free survival compared to TME.[16] A high rate of successful organ-preserving treatment was achieved (88.6%) in their study.

The French GRECCAR 2 randomized 145 patients into local excision vs. total mesorectal excision after neoadjuvant therapy. The most recent update has shown equivalent local recurrence rates (7%), with no difference in overall, disease-free, or cancer-specific mortality. Surgical complications rated were half in the local excision group compared to the TME group after 30 days and nearly 10 times lower after two years. They concluded that local excision is safe and feasible due to the equivalent oncological outcomes.[17]

Quality of life

CRT for rectal cancer is associated with severe acute toxicity that might impair patients' QoL and functioning during and after treatment. Capecitabine has been introduced in the past decade due to its potential benefit compared to continuous intravenous administration of 5-FU, but predominantly because of the convenience to the patient due to the oral availability of capecitabine.[18] During CRT, grade 3 acute toxicity is described in 21.1% of patients with diarrhoea and radiation dermatitis is most prominent.[19] A prospectively conducted observational study described the patient-reported outcomes after CRT in rectal cancer. Just after CRT completion and before any surgery, patients reported worse physical/social functioning, higher levels of fatigue and lower body image.[20] These outcomes recovered to baseline levels 1 year after treatment (90% radical surgery (APR/LAR)).

QoL after local excision versus conventional surgery

An update from the CARTS-study (chemoradiotherapy followed by organ-sparing transanal endoscopic microsurgery (TEM) for distal rectal cancer) described, besides satisfying oncological and organ-preserving outcomes, health-related quality of life in patients with cT1-3N0-1 rectal cancer treated with CRT followed by local excision.[11,21] Patients completed validated questionnaires (EORTC QLQ-C30 and EORTC QLQ-CR38) after an interval of at least 12 months since local excision. An improved emotional functioning was reported in these patients. However, a higher anxiety level was also reported, especially in patients with an incomplete pathological response after TEM surgery. Bowel dysfunction was measured using the LARS questionnaire, resulting in 50% of patients experiencing major LARS after CRT followed by local excision. This is in contrast with outcomes of the EORTC QLQ-C30 questionnaire, where no difference in constipation score and a reduction in diarrhoea score was seen.

Pucciarelli et al. compared quality of life and bowel function in patients with rectal cancer who underwent either local excision or conventional surgery after chemoradiotherapy in a retrospective study.[22] On the functional outcomes scores, patients after local excision reported significantly fewer constipation, sensation of incomplete emptying, and second bowel movements within 15 minutes when compared to the conventional surgery group. On the other hand, there were no differences between the two groups on the functioning scales (physical, role, emotional, cognitive) except for social functioning. The small or absent differences on the generic quality of life questionnaires were explained due to the fact patients report overall health scores that often do not differ from those of the general population.[23] The authors concluded that patients who underwent local excision had a better quality of life and especially bowel function than those who underwent TME.

In the GRECCAR-2 trial, patients diagnosed with cT2-3N0-1 rectal cancer were treated with neoadjuvant chemoradiotherapy and randomized between local excision and conventional TME surgery in case of a good or complete response.[10] At two-year follow-up, there were no differences in morbidity, faecal incontinence, and sexual dysfunction between the local excision and conventional TME surgery groups. The study failed to show superiority of local excision with regard to a composite endpoint of death, recurrence, surgical morbidity, and severe side effects. The absence of this superiority was attributed to the high number of completion TMEs undertaken, which significantly increased the morbidity and complications of the procedure. Thus, adequate preoperative staging remains a key factor, considering the worse outcome following a complete TME.

QoL after local excision versus watch-and-wait strategy

The development of a complete response after chemoradiotherapy has led to the surgical dilemma on how to proceed on this point since a full-thickness local excision or a watch-and-wait policy can be considered. QoL and functional outcomes should be taken into consideration when deciding how to proceed for each patient. In 2016, Habr-Gama et al. published the results of a cohort study with prospectively collected data regarding anorectal manometry and quality of life assessment compared between patients after local excision and a watch-and-wait strategy.[24] Patients with complete clinical response were included in a watch-and-wait strategy, patients with near-complete response (ycT1-2) were managed by transanal endoscopic microsurgery. Although cohort sizes were small and no measurement of baseline manometry, patients after local excision scored worse regarding mean resting pressure, maximal squeeze pressure, and rectal capacity. QoL and functional assessment were performed using the Cleveland Clinic Incontinence Index (CCII) and the Faecal Incontinence

Quality of Life (FIQL) questionnaires. Patients after local excision scored worse on all domains of the CCII (solid stools, liquid stools, gas, use of pads, and lifestyle alterations) as well as on the FIQL domains (lifestyle, coping/behaviour, depression/self-perception and embarrassment). These findings should be taken into consideration for the management of patients after assessment of clinical response to CRT. This study has demonstrated that function preservation seems only achieved with a non-operative management in the setting of a near/complete clinical response.

Future perspectives

The paradigm shift of radical surgery to an organ-sparing treatment for patients with a cCR after CRT is being adapted rapidly worldwide. Long-term oncological outcomes are currently closely monitored in different organ-preserving programmes, and results are being published. Data from prospective studies such as the STAR-TREC study should be awaited before using organ preservation as standard treatment for rectal cancer.[25,26] In the STAR-TREC study two organ preservation arms (chemoradiation or short-course radiotherapy) are randomized and compared to standard TME surgery. Patients with a cCR are observed closely in a watch-and-wait follow-up scheme, whereas patients with a near-complete response are treated with local excision. Patients without a significant response or with high-risk features after local excision or recurrence after watch-and-wait are treated with radical TME surgery. This study is going to demonstrate potential differences in QoL in the organ preservation arms compared to standard TME surgery, but will also demonstrate whether organ preservation is safe with regard to local and distant failures. In order to offer an organ-preserving treatment to rectal cancer patients a clinically significant response is required. To achieve higher rates of cCR optimization of neoadjuvant CRT (nCRT), regimens may be explored to avoid the disadvantage of radical surgery.

Intensified chemoradiotherapy

In 2017, a study from Habr-Gama was published that compared the outcomes of patients diagnosed with cT2N0 distal (<7 cm to anal verge) rectal cancer undergoing standard nCRT versus extended nCRT to demonstrate the potential benefits of more aggressive treatment in terms of organ preservation.[27] Patients undergoing standard CRT (50.4 Gy and two cycles of 5-FU-based chemotherapy) were compared with those undergoing extended CRT (54 Gy and six cycles of 5-FU-based chemotherapy). Clinical complete response rate was significantly higher after extended CRT, 85.7% (30/35 patients) vs. 56.6% (26/46 patients) after standard CRT. Five-year surgery-free survival for all included patients was significantly higher for patients undergoing extended CRT (67% vs. 30%, $p = 0.001$). There were no differences in three-year overall cancer-specific survival between the extended or standard CRT groups (94.0% vs. 94.4%). These data suggest that dose escalation to 54 Gy of radiation and additional cycles of chemotherapy during RT and the resting period may significantly improve the chances of organ preservation for cT2N0 rectal cancer.

Neoadjuvant systemic therapy (FOLFOX in combination with short-course radiotherapy) was studied in the RAPIDO study for advanced tumours and demonstrated an improvement in locoregional control as well as (disease-free) survival. The reported increase in pathological complete response rate for LARC patients undergoing short-course radiotherapy followed by intensified chemotherapy (28%; 120 out of 423 patients) compared to standard care (14%; 57 out of 398 patients) showed its potential when pursuing organ preservation (28). Even more extensive combinations of induction systemic treatment followed by chemoradiation, total neoadjuvant treatment (TNT), is now subject of many studies such as the OPRA study.[29,30] A recent meta-analysis included seven trials focusing on TNT reported an enhanced pCR rate of 29.5% compared to 14.9% with an improved disease-free survival among patients who received TNT.[31] Not only organ preservation, but also toxicity and quality of life with these intensified chemotherapy regimens are to be reported before this will be implemented as a standard treatment option in organ preservation.

High-dose radiotherapy

External beam RT in the combination with additional high-dose-rate endorectal brachytherapy (HDR) might be feasible for patients unfit for chemotherapy or a surgical approach. Appelt et al. showed that a watch-and-wait approach was feasible in 40 of 51 patients after HDR chemoradiotherapy with primary cT2-3N0-1 rectal cancer patients.[32] Local recurrence was observed in 15.5% after one year of follow-up, without any unexpected serious adverse effects. The HERBERT study showed that in unfit LARC patients, radiotherapy followed by HDR resulted in an 88% response rate, with 61% of the patients achieving a clinical CR with acceptable overall survival.[33] These promising results were, unfortunately, accompanied with high rates of significant late toxicity. Nevertheless, elderly, comorbid patients might be candidates for local radiotherapeutic options combined with external beam RT alone or with CRT instead of primary surgical intervention.[34]

X-ray endocavitary brachytherapy (EBRT) already showed to improve local control in T1-2 rectal tumours.[35,36] In recent years, it regained interest for organ preservation strategies. In the Lyon R 96-02 randomized trial, survival benefit did not improve by EBRT, but it led to significantly increased sphincter and organ-sparing rates after 10 years of follow-up.[37] Other reports described that the addition of EBRT enabled rectum preservation in up to 89% of patients staged cT1-3N0 and led to successful sphincter-preserving therapy in 89% of the studied LARC patients.[38,39] The recent OPERA study also demonstrated promising results with (contact) boost therapy following neoadjuvant CRT, aiming for organ preservation.[40] With a reduction of the radiotherapeutic field, higher radiation doses (combined with chemotherapy) can potentially be achieved without severe long-term effects for the healthy tissue.[41–43]

Conclusion

In conclusion, local excision after neoadjuvant treatment can lead to preservation of the rectum and seems an oncologically safe alternative to conventional surgery in patients with a clinically significant or complete response. Patient selection and the assessment of response to neoadjuvant treatment are essential, and strict standardized criteria are recommended. Outcomes in terms of QoL and anorectal function seem to be superior after local excision when compared to conventional surgery but needs further evaluation in prospective trials. Prospective collection of data on an intention-to-treat basis is important to justify neoadjuvant treatment regimens for organ preservation in early rectal cancer patients.[44]

References

1. Lezoche E, Guerrieri M, Paganini AM, Baldarelli M, De Sanctis A, Lezoche G. Long-term results in patients with T2-3 N0 distal rectal cancer undergoing radiotherapy before transanal endoscopic microsurgery. *Br J Surg*. 2005;92(12):1546–52.
2. Kapiteijn E, Marijnen CA, Nagtegaal ID, et al. Preoperative radiotherapy combined with total mesorectal excision for resectable rectal cancer. *N Engl J Med*. 2001;345(9):638–46.
3. Erlandsson J, Holm T, Pettersson D, et al. Optimal fractionation of preoperative radiotherapy and timing to surgery for rectal cancer (Stockholm III): a multicentre, randomised, non-blinded, phase 3, non-inferiority trial. *Lancet Oncol*. 2017;18(3):336–46.
4. Rombouts AJM, Hugen N, Verhoeven RHA, et al. Tumor response after long interval comparing 5x5Gy radiation therapy with chemoradiation therapy in rectal cancer patients. *Eur J Surg Oncol*. 2018;44(7):1018–24.
5. Smart CJ, Korsgen S, Hill J, et al. Multicentre study of short-course radiotherapy and transanal endoscopic microsurgery for early rectal cancer. *Br J Surg*. 2016;103(8):1069–75.
6. Bach SP, Gilbert A, Brock K, et al. Radical surgery versus organ preservation via short-course radiotherapy followed by transanal endoscopic microsurgery for early-stage rectal cancer (TREC): a randomised, open-label feasibility study. *Lancet Gastroenterol Hepatol*. 2021;6(2):92–105.
7. Gilbert A, Homer V, Brock K, et al. Quality-of-life outcomes in older patients with early-stage rectal cancer receiving organ-preserving treatment with hypofractionated short-course radiotherapy followed by transanal endoscopic microsurgery (TREC): non-randomised registry of patients unsuitable for total mesorectal excision. *Lancet Healthy Longev*. 2022;3(12):e825–e38.
8. Habr-Gama A, Perez RO, Nadalin W, et al. Operative versus nonoperative treatment for stage 0 distal rectal cancer following chemoradiation therapy: long-term results. *Ann Surg*. 2004;240(4):711–17; discussion 7–8.
9. Garcia-Aguilar J, Renfro LA, Chow OS, et al. Organ preservation for clinical T2N0 distal rectal cancer using neoadjuvant chemoradiotherapy and local excision (ACOSOG

Z6041): results of an open-label, single-arm, multi-institutional, phase 2 trial. *Lancet Oncol.* 2015;16(15):1537–46.

10. Rullier E, Rouanet P, Tuech JJ, et al. Organ preservation for rectal cancer (GRECCAR 2): a prospective, randomised, open-label, multicentre, phase 3 trial. *Lancet.* 2017;390(10093):469–79.
11. Bokkerink GM, de Graaf EJ, Punt CJ, et al. The CARTS study: Chemoradiation therapy for rectal cancer in the distal rectum followed by organ-sparing transanal endoscopic microsurgery. *BMC Surg.* 2011;11:34.
12. Lezoche G, Baldarelli M, Guerrieri M, et al. A prospective randomized study with a 5-year minimum follow-up evaluation of transanal endoscopic microsurgery versus laparoscopic total mesorectal excision after neoadjuvant therapy. *Surg Endosc.* 2008;22(2):352–8.
13. Shaikh I, Askari A, Ouru S, Warusavitarne J, Athanasiou T, Faiz O. Oncological outcomes of local excision compared with radical surgery after neoadjuvant chemoradiotherapy for rectal cancer: a systematic review and meta-analysis. *Int J Colorectal Dis.* 2015;30(1):19–29.
14. Serra-Aracil X, Pericay C, Badia-Closa J, et al. Short-term outcomes of chemoradiotherapy and local excision versus total mesorectal excision in T2-T3ab,N0,M0 rectal cancer: a multicentre randomised, controlled, phase III trial (the TAU-TEM study). *Ann Oncol.* 2023;34(1):78–90.
15. Maas M, Nelemans PJ, Valentini V, et al. Long-term outcome in patients with a pathological complete response after chemoradiation for rectal cancer: a pooled analysis of individual patient data. *Lancet Oncol.* 2010;11(9):835–44.
16. Creavin B, Ryan E, Martin ST, et al. Organ preservation with local excision or active surveillance following chemoradiotherapy for rectal cancer. *Br J Cancer.* 2017;116(2):169–74.
17. Rullier E, Vendrely V, Asselineau J, et al. Organ preservation with chemoradiotherapy plus local excision for rectal cancer: 5-year results of the GRECCAR 2 randomised trial. *Lancet Gastroenterol Hepatol.* 2020;5(5):465–74.
18. Van Cutsem E, Hoff PM, Harper P, et al. Oral capecitabine vs intravenous 5-fluorouracil and leucovorin: integrated efficacy data and novel analyses from two large, randomised, phase III trials. *Br J Cancer.* 2004;90(6):1190–7.
19. Swellengrebel HA, Marijnen CA, Verwaal VJ, et al. Toxicity and complications of preoperative chemoradiotherapy for locally advanced rectal cancer. *Br J Surg.* 2011;98(3):418–26.
20. Pucciarelli S, Del Bianco P, Efficace F, et al. Patient-reported outcomes after neoadjuvant chemoradiotherapy for rectal cancer: a multicenter prospective observational study. *Ann Surg.* 2011;253(1):71–7.
21. Stijns RCH, de Graaf EJR, Punt CJA, et al. Long-term oncological and functional outcomes of chemoradiotherapy followed by organ-sparing transanal endoscopic microsurgery for distal rectal cancer: the CARTS study. *JAMA Surg.* 2019;154(1):47–54.
22. Pucciarelli S, Giandomenico F, De Paoli A, et al. Bowel function and quality of life after local excision or total mesorectal excision following chemoradiotherapy for rectal cancer. *Br J Surg.* 2017;104(1):138–47.
23. Giandomenico F, Gavaruzzi T, Lotto L, et al. Quality of life after surgery for rectal cancer: a systematic review of comparisons with the general population. *Expert Rev Gastroenterol Hepatol.* 2015;9(9):1227–42.
24. Habr-Gama A, Lynn PB, Jorge JM, et al. Impact of organ-preserving strategies on anorectal function in patients with distal rectal cancer following neoadjuvant chemoradiation. *Dis Colon Rectum.* 2016;59(4):264–9.
25. Rombouts AJM, Al-Najami I, Abbott NL, et al. Can we Save the rectum by watchful waiting or TransAnal microsurgery following (chemo) Radiotherapy versus Total mesorectal excision for early REctal Cancer (STAR-TREC study)?: protocol for a multicentre, randomised feasibility study. *BMJ Open.* 2017;7(12):e019474.

26. Bach SP, Collaborative S-T. Can we Save the rectum by watchful waiting or TransAnal surgery following (chemo)Radiotherapy versus Total mesorectal excision for early REctal Cancer (STAR-TREC)? Protocol for the international, multicentre, rolling phase II/III partially randomized patient preference trial evaluating long-course concurrent chemoradiotherapy versus short-course radiotherapy organ preservation approaches. *Colorectal Dis.* 2022;24(5):639–51.
27. Habr-Gama A, Sao Juliao GP, Vailati BB, et al. Organ preservation in cT2N0 rectal cancer after neoadjuvant chemoradiation therapy: the impact of radiation therapy dose-escalation and consolidation chemotherapy. *Ann Surg.* 2019;269(1):102–7.
28. Bahadoer RR, Dijkstra EA, van Etten B, et al. Short-course radiotherapy followed by chemotherapy before total mesorectal excision (TME) versus preoperative chemoradiotherapy, TME, and optional adjuvant chemotherapy in locally advanced rectal cancer (RAPIDO): a randomised, open-label, phase 3 trial. *Lancet Oncol.* 2021;22(1):29–42.
29. Verheij FS, Omer DM, Williams H, et al. Long-term results of organ preservation in patients with rectal adenocarcinoma treated with total neoadjuvant therapy: the randomized phase II OPRA trial. *J Clin Oncol.* 2023;42(5):500–6.
30. Garcia-Aguilar J, Patil S, Gollub MJ, et al. Organ preservation in patients with rectal adenocarcinoma treated with total neoadjuvant therapy. *J Clin Oncol.* 2022;40(23):2546–56.
31. Kasi A, Abbasi S, Handa S, et al. Total neoadjuvant therapy vs standard therapy in locally advanced rectal cancer: a systematic review and meta-analysis. *JAMA Netw Open.* 2020;3(12):e2030097.
32. Appelt AL, Ploen J, Harling H, et al. High-dose chemoradiotherapy and watchful waiting for distal rectal cancer: a prospective observational study. *Lancet Oncol.* 2015;16(8):919–27.
33. Rijkmans EC, Cats A, Nout RA, et al. Endorectal brachytherapy boost after external beam radiation therapy in elderly or medically inoperable patients with rectal cancer: primary outcomes of the phase 1 HERBERT study. *Int J Radiat Oncol Biol Phys.* 2017;98(4):908–17.
34. Dhadda AS, Martin A, Killeen S, Hunter IA. Organ preservation using contact radiotherapy for early rectal cancer: outcomes of patients treated at a single centre in the UK. *Clin Oncol (R Coll Radiol).* 2017;29(3):198–204.
35. Gerard JP, Chapet O, Ramaioli A, Romestaing P. Long-term control of T2–T3 rectal adenocarcinoma with radiotherapy alone. *Int J Radiat Oncol Biol Phys.* 2002;54(1):142–9.
36. Myerson RJ, Hunt SR. Conservative alternatives to extirpative surgery for rectal cancer. *Clin Oncol (R Coll Radiol).* 2007;19(9):682–6.
37. Ortholan C, Romestaing P, Chapet O, Gerard JP. Correlation in rectal cancer between clinical tumor response after neoadjuvant radiotherapy and sphincter or organ preservation: 10-year results of the Lyon R 96–02 randomized trial. *Int J Radiat Oncol Biol Phys.* 2012;83(2):e165–71.
38. Frin AC, Evesque L, Gal J, et al. Organ or sphincter preservation for rectal cancer. The role of contact X-ray brachytherapy in a monocentric series of 112 patients. *Eur J Cancer.* 2017;72:124–36.
39. Smith FM, Al-Amin A, Wright A, Berry J, Nicoll JJ, Sun Myint A. Contact radiotherapy boost in association with 'watch and wait' for rectal cancer: initial experience and outcomes from a shared programme between a district general hospital network and a regional oncology centre. *Colorectal Dis.* 2016;18(9):861–70.
40. Gerard JP, Barbet N, Schiappa R, et al. Neoadjuvant chemoradiotherapy with radiation dose escalation with contact x-ray brachytherapy boost or external beam radiotherapy boost for organ preservation in early cT2-cT3 rectal adenocarcinoma (OPERA): a phase 3, randomised controlled trial. *Lancet Gastroenterol Hepatol.* 2023;8(4):356–67.
41. Gerard JP, Romestaing P, Chapet O. Radiotherapy alone in the curative treatment of rectal carcinoma. *Lancet Oncol.* 2003;4(3):158–66.

42. Gerard JP, Chapet O, Nemoz C, et al. Improved sphincter preservation in low rectal cancer with high-dose preoperative radiotherapy: the lyon R96-02 randomized trial. *J Clin Oncol.* 2004;22(12):2404–9.
43. Jakobsen A, Ploen J, Vuong T, Appelt A, Lindebjerg J, Rafaelsen SR. Dose-effect relationship in chemoradiotherapy for locally advanced rectal cancer: a randomized trial comparing two radiation doses. *Int J Radiat Oncol Biol Phys.* 2012;84(4):949–54.
44. de Wilt JHW, Bach SP. Is it time for a paradigm shift in early rectal cancer treatment? *Ann Oncol.* 2023;34(4):336–8.

10
Salvage resections post organ preservation for locally advanced rectal cancer

Barbara Noiret, Vincent Assenat, Marc-Olivier François, and Quentin Denost

Introduction

The widespread use of population screening programmes in colorectal cancer has currently increased the number of newly diagnosed early rectal cancer T1–T2 each year.[1] Local excision of early rectal cancer by either transanal endoscopic microsurgery (TEM) or transanal minimally invasive surgery (TAMIS) has become an accepted treatment in selected patients, with the advantages of decreasing both postoperative morbidity and impairment of quality of life. Two different circumstances may lead to TME after local excision.[2] Firstly, the finding of unfavourable features in histopathology, requiring a 'completion TME', and secondly, the occurrence of local recurrence after local excision, requiring 'salvage TME'. Finally, completion and salvage TME have to be considered in two different situations according to the use or not of neoadjuvant chemoradiotherapy before local excision.[3] We will develop in this chapter the indications of TME after local excision, and the consequences of prior local excision followed by completion or salvage TME on postoperative morbidity, functional, and oncological outcomes.

Anatomical considerations

This point is rarely reported in the literature but the location of a tumour has an important impact on the quality of completion or salvage TME (Fig. 10.1). Indeed, in posterior locations, the fat tissue of the mesorectum will protect the TME plane, whereas in anterior locations and in tumours located within 1–2 cm above the anal ring, the mesorectum is lacking and the TME plane may be disrupted by the previous local excision leading to a higher risk of specimen perforation and pelvic sepsis.

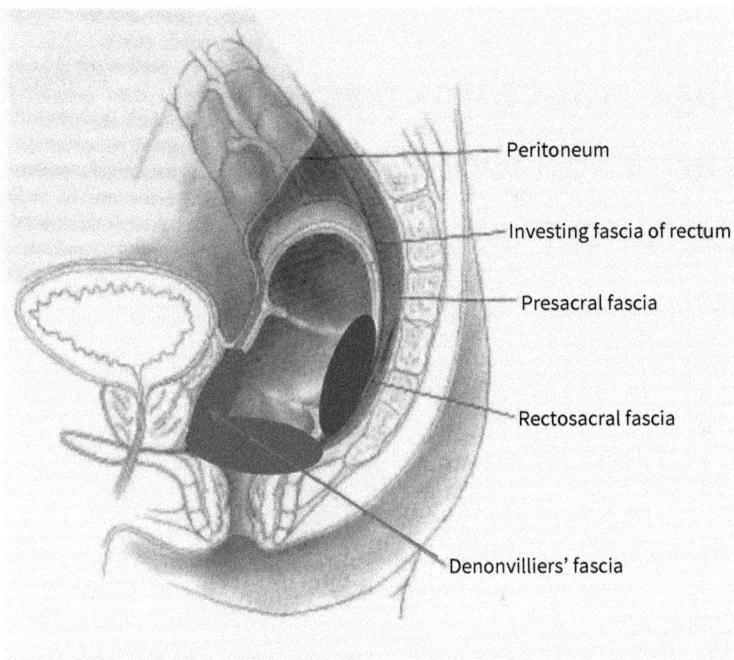

Fig. 10.1 Impact of the location of local excision.

Completion TME

Patients with low-risk T1 carcinomas (well to moderately differentiated, no lymphatic, venous, or perineural invasion, non-mucinous component, diameter less than 3 cm and a clear resection margin) are considered to have an acceptable oncological outcome after local excision without further treatment (Table 10.1).[4–6] If one or more risk factors are present, local recurrence rates of up to 25% have been reported, so completion TME is recommended by many national treatment guidelines.[7–11] Concerning patient innocent of pelvic radiotherapy, recent studies show no difference in terms of surgical morbidity after completion TME compared to primary TME, but an indisputable prolongation of operating time.[12,13]

In contrast, in GRECCAR 2,[14] all patients received chemoradiotherapy before local excision, the absence of superiority of a local excision group compared to the TME group in good responders after chemoradiotherapy was due to a high number of completion TME undertaken, which significantly increased the morbidity and complications of the procedure and therefore compromised the potential advantages of local excision. This increased morbidity is due to the morbidity of completion TME being twice as high after a primary TME. The higher morbidity due to completion TME found in GRECCAR 2 can be the result of additional effects of recent pelvic radiation and local excision.

Table 10.1 Appropriate tumour selection for local excision

Characteristics	Favourable	Unfavourable
1	Well differentiated	Poorly differentiated
2	Moderately differentiated	
3	No lymphovascular invasion	Lymphovascular invasion
4	No perineural invasion	Perineural invasion
5	No mucinous components	Evidence of mucin production
6	Invasion to level sm1 and sm2 <3 cm in size <1/3 the circumference of the rectal wall <10 cm from the anal verge	Invasion to level sm1 and sm3 >3 cm in size >1/3 the circumference of the rectal wall >10 cm from the anal verge
7	Mobile lesion	Fixed lesion

sm, submucosa; cm, centimetre

Sourced from (6) Heafer et al., *J Gastrointest Oncol.* 2014.

If the morbidity does not increase, functional outcome can be compromised with a higher risk of definitive colostomies for patients who underwent completion TME. This is easily explained by a more difficult surgery procedure caused by recent violation of surgical planes, mesorectum fibrotic scar, or weakness of rectal wall due to the TEM. Difficulties in pelvic dissection result in more APR procedures to ensure a safe and radical resection.[3,15]

Moreover, the risk of a poorer quality of mesorectum is real. Operative difficulties can lead to an incomplete specimen with a mesorectal defect in the prior site of local excision especially when full-thickness excisions were previously performed in anterior and distal mesorectum (Fig. 10.1). Even if the impact of a specimen without any tumour left is unknown, the powerful correlation between specimen's quality and oncological outcome is certain, completion TME after local excision doesn't impair the oncological prognosis in term of local recurrence rate and overall survival but reduces the disease-free survival for patients with a poorer specimen.[1,2,16,17]

Salvage TME

Salvage TME is used with curative intent after a local recurrence following a prior local excision for early rectal cancer. Recurrence rates after LE for low-risk carcinoma are between 10% and 20% according to several studies and median time for recurrence is 15 months.[2] Salvage surgery can allow a R0 resection in the majority of cases at the cost of preoperative treatment by chemoradiotherapy to ensure free margins before surgical resection.[6]

Local recurrence is usually endo-luminal but can also occur with larger pelvic invasion. Indeed, current methods of surveillance can miss microscopic recurrence at an early stage with extensive local recurrence being encountered due to this. In these cases, classic TME won't always be efficient and a larger pelvic exenteration could be necessary with higher morbidity and poor functional outcomes due to less sphincteric preservation. The need to perform an extended pelvic resection is also correlated with poorer oncological outcome.[18] Overall survival and functional outcomes are better for endo-luminal recurrence than pelvic ones.[19]

Some patients are not eligible for salvage TME due to comorbidities. Some patients undergo local re-excision followed by systemic chemotherapy; however, very poor oncological outcomes and a low five-year survival rate compared to salvage TME are seen. This confirms that even if results in terms of functional and oncological outcomes are disappointing according to the initial early disease stage, salvage TME remains the best treatment of local recurrence post local excision.[20]

Advantages of the TaTME approach for TME post local excision

Completion TME must include the entire prior resection site. As noted previously, it can be a difficult procedure due to fibrotic changes and pelvic adhesions induced by previous TEM. These difficulties lead to more radical resection to the detriment of functional outcomes and increase the risk of producing a poorer specimen with worse oncological outcomes. Transanal TME is a good solution to get around complications and produce an intact specimen, avoiding perforation into the operating field. TaTME dissection is performed under direct visualization allowing a more precise approach to TEM's scar.

Dissection is led by both sides with less traction on the mesorectum reducing the risk of plane disruption and rectal perforation especially when previous local excision has been done in the distal mesorectum. Indeed, in these conditions, APRs were frequently chosen to ensure a good quality of specimen, imposing a definitive stoma.[15] Transanal approach is a great alternative, improving the accuracy of TME dissection and avoiding definitive colostomy. Compared to classic completion TME, completion TaTME leads to better functional results with a lower rate of definitive stoma and improves safety and quality of the mesorectal dissection.[21]

Conclusion

Total mesorectum excision remains the gold standard for rectal cancer treatment. However, full-thickness local excision has incontestable benefit over TME in terms of bowel, urinary, and sexual function, but also concerning cost and hospital stay for early rectal cancer management. Unfortunately, preoperative staging is not always able to distinguish T1 from T2 cancer and to identify risk factors of recurrence, such as lymphatic, venous, or perineural invasion. When bad prognosis factors are present, local excision can be regarded as staging a big biopsy and has to be followed by a completion TME, which remains the gold standard compared to a general treatment alone.[20,22]

Due to several operative difficulties after local excision, completion TME has acceptable oncological results, but gives poor functional results compared to a primary TME, which is why in these conditions TaTME has a good indication to overcome these operative difficulties.

Salvage surgery after local recurrence can, most of the time, ensure a free resection margin but long-term oncological outcomes are poor. It emphasizes that the selection of patients treated by local excision for early rectal cancer must be highly rigorous.

References

1. Stamos MJ, Murrell Z. Management of early rectal T1 and T2 cancers. *Clin Cancer Res.* 2007;13(22 Pt 2):6885s–9s.
2. Jones HJS, Cunningham C, Nicholson GA, Hompes R. Outcomes following completion and salvage surgery for early rectal cancer: a systematic review. *Eur J Surg Oncol.* 2018;44(1):15–23.
3. van Gijn W, Brehm V, de Graaf E, et al. Unexpected rectal cancer after TEM: outcome of completion surgery compared with primary TME. *Eur J Surg Oncol.* 2013;39(11):1225–9.
4. Bosch SL, Teerenstra S, de Wilt JHW, Cunningham C, Nagtegaal ID. Predicting lymph node metastasis in pT1 colorectal cancer: a systematic review of risk factors providing rationale for therapy decisions. *Endoscopy.* 2013;45(10):827–34.
5. Bach SP, Hill J, Monson JRT, et al. A predictive model for local recurrence after transanal endoscopic microsurgery for rectal cancer. *Br J Surg.* 2009;96(3):280–90.
6. Heafner TA, Glasgow SC. A critical review of the role of local excision in the treatment of early (T1 and T2) rectal tumors. *J Gastrointest Oncol.* 2014;5(5):345–52.
7. Peeters KCMJ, van de Velde CJH, Leer JWH, et al. Late side effects of short-course preoperative radiotherapy combined with total mesorectal excision for rectal cancer: increased bowel dysfunction in irradiated patients—a Dutch colorectal cancer group study. *J Clin Oncol.* 2005;23(25):6199–206.
8. Rutten HJT, den Dulk M, Lemmens VEPP, van de Velde CJH, Marijnen CAM. Controversies of total mesorectal excision for rectal cancer in elderly patients. *Lancet Oncol.* 2008;9(5):494–501.
9. Swellengrebel HAM, Marijnen CAM, Verwaal VJ, et al. Toxicity and complications of preoperative chemoradiotherapy for locally advanced rectal cancer. *Br J Surg.* 2011;98(3):418–26.
10. Hompes R, Cunningham C. Extending the role of transanal endoscopic microsurgery (TEM) in rectal cancer. *Colorectal Dis.* 2011;13 Suppl 7:32–6.
11. Oncoline. Richtlijnen. 2022. https://www.oncoline.nl/colorectaalcarcinoom
12. Coton C, Lefevre JH, Debove C, et al. Does transanal local resection increase morbidity for subsequent total mesorectal excision for early rectal cancer? *Colorectal Dis.* 2019;21(1):15–22.

13. Eid Y, Alves A, Lubrano J, Menahem B. Does previous transanal excision for early rectal cancer impair surgical outcomes and pathologic findings of completion total mesorectal excision? Results of a systematic review of the literature. *J Visc Surg*. 2018;155(6):445–52.
14. Rullier E, Vendrely V, Asselineau J, et al. Organ preservation with chemoradiotherapy plus local excision for rectal cancer: 5-year results of the GRECCAR 2 randomised trial. *Lancet Gastroenterol Hepatol*. 5(5):465–74.
15. Morino M, Allaix ME, Arolfo S, Arezzo A. Previous transanal endoscopic microsurgery for rectal cancer represents a risk factor for an increased abdominoperineal resection rate. *Surg Endosc*. 2013;27(9):3315–21.
16. Hahnloser D, Wolff BG, Larson DW, Ping J, Nivatvongs S. Immediate radical resection after local excision of rectal cancer: an oncologic compromise? *Dis Colon Rectum*. 2005;48(3):429–37.
17. Hompes R, McDonald R, Buskens C, et al. Completion surgery following transanal endoscopic microsurgery: assessment of quality and short- and long-term outcome. *Colorectal Dis*. 2013;15(10):e576–81.
18. Bikhchandani J, Ong GK, Dozois EJ, Mathis KL. Outcomes of salvage surgery for cure in patients with locally recurrent disease after local excision of rectal cancer. *Dis Colon Rectum*. 2015;58(3):283–7.
19. Weiser MR, Landmann RG, Wong WD, et al. Surgical salvage of recurrent rectal cancer after transanal excision. *Dis Colon Rectum*. 2005;48(6):1169–75.
20. Stipa F, Giaccaglia V, Burza A. Management and outcome of local recurrence following transanal endoscopic microsurgery for rectal cancer. *Dis Colon Rectum*. 2012;55(3):262–9.
21. Koedam TWA, Veltcamp Helbach M, Penna M, et al. Short-term outcomes of transanal completion total mesorectal excision (cTaTME) for rectal cancer: a case-matched analysis. *Surg Endosc*. 2019;33(1):103–9.
22. Borstlap WAA, Tanis PJ, Koedam TWA, et al. A multi-centred randomised trial of radical surgery versus adjuvant chemoradiotherapy after local excision for early rectal cancer. *BMC Cancer*. 2016;16:513.

11
Follow-up protocols for rectal cancer patients undergoing organ preservation

Jan Žmuc and Geerard L. Beets

Introduction

At present, the standard treatment for nonmetastatic rectal cancer is radical surgical resection combined with chemoradiotherapy (CRT) for advanced disease stages. The main aim of follow-up is to improve survival through early detection and curative treatment of both local recurrences and distant metastases, as well as the detection of new primary colorectal cancers. Additional aims of follow-up are improving quality of life through early discovery and management of late treatment complications and collection of treatment outcome data for quality audit and research purposes. Whether intensive surveillance after treatment for colorectal cancer results in improved survival is controversial.[1] Nevertheless, there is a general consensus among expert groups that patients after resection of rectal cancer should undergo regular clinical examination, serum carcinoembryonic antigen level measurement, flexible endoscopy, and CT imaging for at least five years.[2]

Approximately 20% of patients with rectal cancer have a complete response to CRT, with no detectable tumour cells in resected specimens. Complete responses are associated with a favourable prognosis, questioning the need for radical rectal resection.[3] The organ preservation approach has repeatedly been shown to be feasible and safe. The majority of patients initially treated non-operatively avoided radical surgery, almost all of the local regrowths were detected early and successfully salvaged, and most studies reported no difference in survival.[4–7] A consensus regarding the terminology has also been achieved, with the term regrowth being used to describe intraluminal or mesorectal recurrence after organ preservation.[8]

Regrowths after organ preservation should be detected and treated early to ensure comparable oncologic outcomes to standard treatment with radical surgery. Most regrowths occur in the first two years post-CRT and intensive surveillance of organ preservation patients in this time period has been recommended.[9] However, the optimal follow-up schedule has not yet been determined. The purpose of this chapter is to review and summarize the available systematic evidence for follow-up after organ preservation and to discuss possible future developments.

Review of follow-up protocols for organ preservation

A literature search was performed using a strategy similar to those described by recent meta-analyses and systematic reviews on non-operative management of rectal cancer.[4–6] We extracted the data from relevant studies to determine what additional investigations were done in organ preservation patients in addition to the standard rectal cancer follow-up protocol outlined in the introduction of this chapter. We excluded studies with overlapping patient cohorts and studies that did not report clear and unambiguous follow-up protocols from our analysis. The results are presented in Table 11.1 for the seven (partially) prospective studies and in Table 11.2 for the nine retrospective studies we included in our analysis.[10–25]

The main finding of this short review is that the included patients were mostly re-examined every three months the first year of follow-up, every three to six months the second year, and twice yearly from years three to five. The most common duration of follow-up was five years.[10,13,14,16,17,23,25] Patients were followed for longer than five years in three of the included studies.[12,21,22] Several studies did not specify the predicted total duration of follow-up.[11,18,19,24] The studies by Renehan et al. and Sanchez Loria et al. reported intensive follow-up for organ preservation patients only for the first two years, with standard surveillance afterwards.[15,20]

Digital rectal exam (DRE) was combined with endoscopy in almost all of the studies, as only Seshadri et al. used endoscopy selectively for suspected recurrences.[21] Regular imaging during follow-up was more prevalent in the prospective studies.

Table 11.1 Reported follow-up intervals in prospective studies

	Year 1			Year 2			Year 3			Year 4 and 5		
First author	DRE/ endo	MRI	PET-CT	DRE/ endo	MRI	PET-CT	DRE/ endo	MRI	PET-CT	DRE/ endo	MRI	PET-CT
Appelt et al.	2		4	3		6	6		12	12		12
Creavin et al.	3–6	3–6		3–6	3–6		3–6	3–6		3–6	3–6	
Habr-Gama et al.	2	6*	6*	3–4	6*	6*	6	12*	12*	6		
Martens et al.	3	3		6	6		6	6		6	6	
Nahas et al.	3	3		3	6		3	6		6	6	
Renehan et al.^	4–6	4–6		4–6	4–6							
Sposato et al.	3–6	6		3–6	6		6	6		6	6	

^ Partially retrospective; * either MRI or PET-CT was performed. All values in months

Table 11.2 Reported follow-up intervals in retrospective studies

	Year 1			Year 2			Year 3			Year 4 and 5		
First author	DRE/ endo	MRI	PET-CT	DRE/ endo	MRI	PET-CT	DRE/ endo	MRI	PET-CT	DRE/ endo	MRI	PET-CT
Araujo et al.	3			3			6			6		
Lai et al.	3	6		3	12		6	12		6	12	
Park et al.	3			3			6			6		
Sanchez Loria et al.	3	3		3	3							
Seshadri et al.	1			3			3			6		
Smith et al. (2015)	3		6	6		12	6		12	12		12
Smith et al. (2019)	3			4			6			6		
Strode et al.	3–4			3–4			4–6			4–6		
Yeom et al.	3			3			6			6		

All values in months

MRI was more commonly used than PET-CT, as it was routinely used in seven of the included studies. PET-CT was routinely used in studies by Appelt et al. and Smith et al. (2015), while Habr-Gama et al. reported using both PET-CT and MRI during follow-up.[10,12,22]

Discussion of current follow-up protocols and future perspectives

Follow-up investigations

At present, there is little data available on which diagnostic investigation is the most successful at detecting regrowths. The studies included in our review most commonly used DRE, endoscopy, and MRI for this purpose. The same investigations are used to accurately assess response and look for residual tumour after CRT.[26] Nearly all of the included studies used regular DRE and endoscopy during follow-up, with just one study omitting routine endoscopic surveillance in favour of an as-needed approach in case of suspected regrowths.[21] This is not surprising, as van der Valk et al. reported that 97% of regrowths are located in the bowel wall and thus can be detected by DRE and endoscopy.[9] The included studies often used standardized DRE and endoscopic response criteria proposed by Habr-Gama et al. to distinguish between benign post-CRT changes and suspected regrowths.[27] Typical changes associated with complete responses are a smooth bowel wall with a subtle loss of pliability felt on DRE and a flat white scar seen on endoscopy. None of the studies included in our review used regular biopsies of post-CRT mucosal changes to detect regrowths, as this approach has been shown to have poor negative predictive value for excluding residual disease.[28] However, abnormal findings such as ulceration, palpable nodules, or stenosis are associated with regrowths. Biopsies should be taken from suspected regrowths to try and histologically confirm cancer recurrence before proceeding with additional treatment.[27] Benign-looking adenomatous lesions will also sometimes be observed during follow-up in organ preservation patients. These may have been the origin of invasive cancer, which disappeared after CRT. Benign-looking lesions should also be biopsied, and if no invasive cancer is found, removed with local excision.[29]

The main limitations of DRE and endoscopy in follow-up of organ preservation patients are the inability to detect regrowths outside of the rectal lumen, either located deep in the rectal wall or in the mesorectum (i.e. lymph nodes or extramural venous invasion).[26,30] All of the prospective studies included in our review have used additional imaging to improve regrowth detection outside of the lumen.[10–16] Additional imaging was less often used in the included retrospective studies, with the caveat that the reported follow-up protocols maybe did not contain inconsistent imaging practices.[17–23] Pelvic MRI was found to be the most commonly used additional imaging investigation in our review. This was expected, as the use of MRI with the addition of diffusion-weighted imaging has been shown to improve the detection of small regrowths after CRT.[31] Among studies included in our review, PET-CT was less commonly used for follow-up. One possible reason is that PET-CT reportedly has lower sensitivity and negative predictive value for detecting complete responses after CRT in comparison to MRI.[32] Therefore, PET-CT could also be less accurate in detecting regrowths. Other possible reasons are that the routine use of PET-CT during follow-up exposes patients to high doses of ionizing radiation, and the higher cost of PET-CT. None of the included studies routinely used other imaging modalities such as endoluminal ultrasound for follow-up of organ preservation patients.

Intervals and duration of follow-up

What is also unclear at present is how often and for how long the organ preservation-specific follow-up is needed. In their analysis of data for 880 patients from the International Watch & Wait Database, van der Valk et al. reported that 88% of all regrowths were diagnosed in the first two years of follow-up.[9] These findings are important, as they seem to hint at the possibility of reducing the intensity of follow-up for organ preservation patients after two years, as the majority of regrowths will occur in that time period. Indeed, two of the studies included in our review already reported only a two-year organ preservation follow-up protocol.[15,20] Another possible optimization of follow-up, according to the data published by van der Valk et al., would be a reduction in the use of costly imaging while continuing endoscopic follow-up, as the vast majority of regrowths occurred in the bowel wall and therefore could be detected by endoscopy.[9]

One of the main criticisms of the organ preservation approach is the presumed cost-inefficiency of the required intensive follow-up.[33] This is probably due to the fact that current organ preservation follow-up protocols emphasized oncological safety and regrowth detection over reducing invasiveness and optimizing cost. Furthermore, the current scarcity of data on regrowth timing and localization precludes the identification and elimination of low-yield and cost-inefficient follow-up examinations. Despite this, a recent paper by Gani et al. found that even current approaches to non-operative management of rectal cancer (with 15 additional pelvic MRIs and rectoscopies during a five-year follow-up period) should be more cost-efficient than immediate radical surgery. In their analysis, non-operative management resulted in lower costs even when simulated for a 25% regrowth rate with included costs of subsequent salvage surgery.[33] The predicted 25% regrowth rate corresponds to the two-year cumulative incidence of regrowths reported by van der Valk et al.[9]

One additional challenge of developing a robust and efficient follow-up protocol for organ preservation is the major difference in risk of recurrence between different subgroups of organ preservation patients. Chadi et al. and Habr-Gama et al. reported that patients with cT3–4 tumours have an increased risk of local regrowth, which could warrant more intensive follow-up in this patient subgroups.[34,35] Interestingly, Habr-Gama et al. also found that baseline node-positive patients do not seem to have more regrowths than node-negative patients, which should obviate the need for additional imaging in node-positive patients.[36] Another organ preservation subgroup which might require a tailored approach to follow-up are the patients who achieve organ preservation through intensified local treatment such as local excision or a contact radiotherapy boost.[37,38] A substantial number of these patients would not have had a complete response with standard CRT regimens, and therefore have a higher risk for harbouring residual disease in regional lymph nodes. These patients may require a follow-up protocol with more frequent MRI imaging than the patients who achieve a complete clinical response after standard CRT.

Conclusion

At present, follow-up in organ preservation patients is performed with a combination of DRE, endoscopy, and MRI. The investigations are repeated every three to six months for the first two years of follow-up, as most regrowths occur within this time period. The usual duration of organ preservation follow-up is five years. Current follow-up protocols are not evidence based. However, the accumulating data from clinical studies and international patient registries on regrowth timing, localization, and detection are expected to optimize follow-up by reducing low-yield or cost-inefficient diagnostic investigations.

References

1. Wille-Jørgensen P, Syk I, Smedh K, et al. Effect of more vs less frequent follow-up testing on overall and colorectal cancer-specific mortality in patients with stage II or III colorectal cancer the COLOFOL randomized clinical trial. *JAMA*. 2018;319(20):2095–103.
2. Luzietti E, Pellino G, Nikolaou S, et al. Comparison of guidelines for the management of rectal cancer. *BJS Open*. 2018;2(6):433–51.
3. Maas M, Nelemans PJ, Valentini V, et al. Long-term outcome in patients with a pathological complete response after chemoradiation for rectal cancer: a pooled analysis of individual patient data. *Lancet Oncol*. 2010;11(9):835–44.
4. Dossa F, Chesney TR, Acuna SA, Baxter NN. A watch-and-wait approach for locally advanced rectal cancer after a clinical complete response following neoadjuvant chemoradiation: a systematic review and meta-analysis. *Lancet Gastroenterol Hepatol*. 2017;2:501–13.
5. Sammour T, Price BA, Krause KJ, Chang GJ. Nonoperative management or 'watch and wait' for rectal cancer with complete clinical response after neoadjuvant chemoradiotherapy: a critical appraisal. *Ann Surg Oncol*. 2017;24(7):1904–15.
6. Dattani M, Heald RJ, Goussous G, et al. Oncological and survival outcomes in Watch and Wait patients with a clinical complete response after neoadjuvant chemoradiotherapy for rectal cancer a systematic review and pooled analysis. *Ann Surg*. 2018;268(6):955–67.
7. Kong JC, Guerra GR, Warrier SK, Ramsay RG, Heriot AG. Outcome and salvage surgery following 'watch and wait' for rectal cancer after neoadjuvant therapy: a systematic review. *Dis Colon Rectum*. 2017;60(3):335–45.
8. Heald RJ, Beets G, Carvalho C. Report from a consensus meeting: Response to chemoradiotherapy in rectal cancer—predictor of cure and a crucial new choice for the patient: on behalf of the Champalimaud 2014 Faculty for 'Rectal cancer: When NOT to operate'. *Color Dis*. 2014;16(5):334–7.
9. van der Valk MJM, Hilling DE, Bastiaannet E, et al. Long-term outcomes of clinical complete responders after neoadjuvant treatment for rectal cancer in the International Watch & Wait Database (IWWD): an international multicentre registry study. *Lancet*. 2018;391(10139):2537–45.
10. Appelt AL, Pløen J, Harling H, et al. High-dose chemoradiotherapy and watchful waiting for distal rectal cancer: a prospective observational study. *Lancet Oncol*. 2015;16(8):919–27.
11. Creavin B, Ryan E, Martin ST, et al. Organ preservation with local excision or active surveillance following chemoradiotherapy for rectal cancer. *Br J Cancer*. 2017;116(2):169–74.
12. Habr-Gama A, Sabbaga J, Gama-Rodrigues J, et al. Watch and wait approach following extended neoadjuvant chemoradiation for distal rectal cancer: are we getting closer to anal cancer management? *Dis Colon Rectum*. 2013;56(10):1109–17.
13. Martens MH, Maas M, Heijnen LA, et al. Long-term outcome of an organ preservation program after neoadjuvant treatment for rectal cancer. *J Natl Cancer Inst*. 2016;108(12):1–10.
14. Nahas SC, Rizkallah Nahas CS, Sparapan Marques CF, et al. Pathologic complete response in rectal cancer: can we detect it? lessons learned from a proposed randomized trial of watch-and-wait treatment of rectal cancer. *Dis Colon Rectum*. 2016;59(4):255–63.
15. Renehan AG, Malcomson L, Emsley R, et al. Watch-and-wait approach versus surgical resection after chemoradiotherapy for patients with rectal cancer (the OnCoRe project): A propensity-score matched cohort analysis. *Lancet Oncol*. 2016;17(2):174–83.
16. Sposato LA, Lam Y, Karapetis C, et al. Observation of 'complete clinical response' in rectal cancer after neoadjuvant chemoradiation: the Flinders experience. *Asia Pac J Clin Oncol*. 2018;14(6):439–45.

17. Araujo ROC, Valadão M, Borges D, et al. Nonoperative management of rectal cancer after chemoradiation opposed to resection after complete clinical response. A comparative study. *Eur J Surg Oncol.* 2015;41(11):1456–63.
18. Lai CL, Lai MJ, Wu CC, Jao SW, Hsiao CW. Rectal cancer with complete clinical response after neoadjuvant chemoradiotherapy, surgery, or 'watch and wait'. *Int J Colorectal Dis.* 2016;31(2):413–19.
19. Park IJ, Lee JL, Yoon YS, et al. Oncologic outcomes of organ preserving approaches in patients with rectal cancer treated with preoperative chemoradiotherapy. *Ann Coloproctol.* 2019;35(2):65–71.
20. Sanchez Loria F, Iseas S, O'Connor JM, et al. Non-surgical management of rectal cancer. Series of 68 cases, long follow up in two leading centres in Argentina. *Dig Liver Dis.* 2016;48(11):1372–7.
21. Seshadri RA, Kondaveeti SS, Jayanand SB, et al. Complete clinical response to neoadjuvant chemoradiation in rectal cancers: Can surgery be avoided? *Hepatogastroenterology.* 2013;60:410–14.
22. Smith RK, Fry RD, Mahmoud NN, Paulson EC. Surveillance after neoadjuvant therapy in advanced rectal cancer with complete clinical response can have comparable outcomes to total mesorectal excision. *Int J Colorectal Dis.* 2015;30(6):769–74.
23. Smith JJ, Strombom P, Chow OS, et al. Assessment of a watch-and-wait strategy for rectal cancer in patients with a complete response after neoadjuvant therapy. *JAMA Oncol.* 2019;5(4):1–8.
24. Strode M, Shah R, Boland PM, et al. Nonoperative management after neoadjuvant therapy for rectal cancer: a single institution experience over 5 years. *Surg Oncol.* 2019;28:116–20.
25. Yeom SS, Lee SY, Kim CH, Kim YJ, Nam TK, Kim HR. Non-operative treatment outcome for rectal cancer patient with clinical complete response after neoadjuvant chemoradiotherapy. *Asian J Surg.* 2019;42(8):823–31.
26. Maas M, Lambregts DMJ, Nelemans PJ, et al. Assessment of clinical complete response after chemoradiation for rectal cancer with digital rectal examination, endoscopy, and MRI: selection for organ-saving treatment. *Ann Surg Oncol.* 2015;22(12):3873–80.
27. Habr-Gama A, Perez RO, Wynn G, Marks J, Kessler H, Gama-Rodrigues J. Complete clinical response after neoadjuvant chemoradiation therapy for distal rectal cancer: characterization of clinical and endoscopic findings for standardization. *Dis Colon Rectum.* 2010;53(12):1692–8.
28. Perez RO, Habr-Gama A, Pereira GV, et al. Role of biopsies in patients with residual rectal cancer following neoadjuvant chemoradiation after downsizing: can they rule out persisting cancer? *Color Dis.* 2012;14(6):714–20.
29. Rupinski M, Szczepkowski M, Malinowska M, et al. Watch and wait policy after preoperative radiotherapy for rectal cancer; management of residual lesions that appear clinically benign. *Eur J Surg Oncol.* 2016;42(2):288–96.
30. Duldulao MP, Lee W, Streja L, et al. Distribution of residual cancer cells in the bowel wall after neoadjuvant chemoradiation in patients with rectal cancer. *Dis Colon Rectum.* 2013;56(2):142–9.
31. Lambregts DMJ, Lahaye MJ, Heijnen LA, et al. MRI and diffusion-weighted MRI to diagnose a local tumour regrowth during long-term follow-up of rectal cancer patients treated with organ preservation after chemoradiotherapy. *Eur Radiol.* 2016;26(7):2118–25.
32. Li YL, Wu LM, Chen XX, Delproposto Z, Hu JN, Xu JR. Is diffusion-weighted MRI superior to FDG-PET or FDG-PET/CT in evaluating and predicting pathological response to preoperative neoadjuvant therapy in patients with rectal cancer? *J Dig Dis.* 2014;15(10):525–37.

33. Gani C, Grosse U, Clasen S, et al. Cost analysis of a wait-and-see strategy after radiochemotherapy in distal rectal cancer. *Strahlentherapie und Onkol.* 2018;194(11):985–90.
34. Chadi SA, Malcomson L, Ensor J, et al. Factors affecting local regrowth after watch and wait for patients with a clinical complete response following chemoradiotherapy in rectal cancer (InterCoRe consortium): an individual participant data meta-analysis. *Lancet Gastroenterol Hepatol.* 2018;3(12):825–36.
35. Habr-Gama A, São Julião GP, Gama-Rodrigues J, et al. Baseline T classification predicts early tumor regrowth after nonoperative management in distal rectal cancer after extended neoadjuvant chemoradiation and initial complete clinical response. *Dis Colon Rectum.* 2017;60(6):586–94.
36. Habr-Gama A, São Julião GP, Vailati BB, et al. Organ preservation among patients with clinically node-positive rectal cancer: is it really more dangerous? *Dis Colon Rectum.* 2019;62(6):675–83.
37. Myint AS, Smith FML, Gollins SW, et al. Dose escalation using contact X-ray brachytherapy (Papillon) for rectal cancer: does it improve the chance of organ preservation? *Br J Radiol.* 2017;90(1080):20170175.
38. Arezzo A, Lo Secco G, Passera R, et al. Individual participant data pooled-analysis of risk factors for recurrence after neoadjuvant radiotherapy and transanal local excision of rectal cancer: the PARTTLE study. *Tech Coloproctol.* 2019;23(9):831–42.

12
Organ preservation for curative management of older patients with rectal cancer and in the palliative setting

Éanna J. Ryan, Brenda Murphy, Ben Creavin, and Desmond Winter

Specific considerations for elderly rectal cancer patient management

Half of patients >70 years with rectal cancer will have a cardiovascular comorbidity, while 20% will have had a previous malignancy. There is a higher risk of adverse events with neoadjuvant/adjuvant treatment and an increased risk of morbidity and mortality.[1] However, it is also important to remember that chronological age may not necessarily reflect an individual patient's overall health,[2] and all older patients with rectal cancer should undergo multidisciplinary team (MDT) discussion, including a dedicated frailty assessment to discuss the most appropriate management strategy that reflects their disease, baseline health status, and expressed wishes.[3]

While there has been a global improvement in survival for rectal cancer in recent years, this is not evident in older rectal cancer patients.[4] Rectal cancer-related mortality increases by almost 40% for every half decade >70 years of age.[5] Patients ≥75 years with concomitant cardiovascular and pulmonary disease suffer twice as many adverse events as those without.[6] While anastomotic leak (AL) rates do not differ based on age, AL is fatal in more than half of patients >75 years, compared to <10% in younger cohorts.[7]

Older CRC patients receive less surgery than their younger counterparts, with resection rates falling from 68% in those 64–74 years of age to 40% in patients >80 years. Unfortunately, this is associated with a decreased use of multimodal treatments, precluding a chance for curative LE or a W&W approach.[8] The Bowel Cancer UK Critical Research Gaps in Colorectal Cancer Initiative has also emphasized the requirement for increasing awareness of QoL concerns for those surviving with and beyond their diagnosis in an effort to guarantee optimal outcomes. It also highlights effective two-way communication between doctors and patients, and for older patients to be actively involved in decision-making in relation to their own care. In this way, it is hoped that a balance between treatment-related morbidity, the risk of recurrence and patient preferences may be reached, and over/undertreatment of older patients may be avoided.[9]

Frailty and older rectal cancer patients

Traditionally, surgeons have relied on either arbitrary cut-offs (i.e. age) or on hunch and intuition when identifying high-risk older patients. A patient's cognition, nutritional level, or an accurate morbidity evaluation cannot be surmised in a 'once-off' immediate impression. Multiple studies have shown that in older adults, frailty as defined by validated geriatric tools (e.g. International Society of Geriatric Oncology (SIOG) score), has been deemed a more accurate surgical risk predictor.[10]

Interpretation of the available literature pertaining to the management of older persons with rectal cancer should be done with caution, as the data are either chronologically based or devoid of evidence. The goal of management for this population should be to safely provide potentially curative, life-extending treatment in such a way that allows the patient to return to their baseline functional status in the shortest duration possible. In older patients, an estimation of their performance status is important to reveal frailty, as this may distinguish management strategies for these patients (TME vs. organ preservation). However, surgeons should remain cognizant that only a small percentage of the older population is considered frail, defined as a state of reduced physiological reserve capacity across multiple organ systems.[11] As a result, the capacity to withstand stressors, such as intensive treatment, is reduced, and there is increased risk of treatment-related adverse events, prolonged or re-hospitalization, and diminished survival.[12,13]

For these reasons its paramount to differentiate between the frail and fit older patient, with no single tool demonstrating complete accuracy.[12] Performing a geriatrician-led comprehensive geriatric assessment (CGA) on a routine basis is time-consuming and impractical.[14] Other less time- and resource-intensive tools are required to screen for frailty in daily practice[12]. Emphasis should be placed on recognizing the main predictors of frailty and postoperative complications, such as functional status, exercise tolerance, nutritional status, and comorbidities in order to identify those patients who will benefit most from a CGA by a geriatrician.[12]

Functional status and frailty screening

Functional status may be rapidly assessed with a timed-up-and-go (TUG) test, as a TUG is predictive of increased complications.[15] A detailed falls history should be sought as a fall in the preceding 6 months is associated with increased complications.[14]

Experts recommend using the Geriatric 8 (G8) score to determine overall health, nutritional status and medication use, and the Mini-Cog© Score to screen for cognitive impairment.[12]

Comprehensive geriatric assessment (CGA)

CGA allows the multiple domains of frailty to be assessed by geriatricians, including physical, nutritional, functional and psychosocial health status, cognition, and polypharmacy.[16] Where frailty is present, prehabilitation programmes should be instigated to improve the patient's condition prior to management, or the management should be tailored to the health status.

Exercise tolerance and prehabilitation

Prehabilitation is one proposed strategy to increase the capacity of older patients to tolerate treatment and enhance recovery.[17] Older patients with physical decline have the greatest risk for postoperative complications; therefore, they have the most to benefit from prehabilitation.[13] Multimodal interventions such as physical training, smoking cessation, nutritional support, and psychological support offer the most benefit.[17–19] This should occur during the period between diagnosis and the initiation of management.

Nutritional status

About one-fifth of patients with CRC are malnourished and this is associated with a catabolic state and adverse outcomes,[20] while an optimized nutritional status is important for muscle gain and recovery.[13] When integrated with other prehabilitation modalities, nutritional interventions can be associated with meaningful improvements in clinical outcomes.[21,22]

Optimizing comorbidities

Approximately 60% of CRC patients over 70 years suffer from some comorbidity.[23] Each comorbidity has a different impact on physical function and postoperative outcomes and should be considered in isolation and as part of a cumulative risk. Targeted management should be undertaken prior to selecting an appropriate treatment schedule.[24,25] Most elderly patients with rectal cancer will have cardiovascular and pulmonary comorbidities, which both increase the operative and postoperative risk.[23,26] Neurological conditions also appear to increase the risk of adverse outcomes.[26] Hypertension, diabetes, and previous malignancies have less of an impact on frailty and outcomes.[23,27]

Radiotherapy and chemotherapy in older patients

The feasibility of nCRT in elderly patients depends on patient frailty and comorbidity. Radiation tolerance is contingent on the treatment volume, and in seniors, smaller volumes should be considered. Good tolerance is imperative in elderly frail patients because if toxicity occurs it can very difficult to manage and may be life-threatening. Renal insufficiency may prevent the use of Capecitabine and considerable care should be taken to ensure compliance with oral therapy, especially in patients living by themselves.

In older patients, neoadjuvant short-course radiotherapy (SCRT) may demonstrate some benefit in terms of treatment-related toxicity.[28,29] SCRT followed by neoadjuvant chemotherapy is an option for increasing response rates and decreasing distant recurrence but tolerance in elderly patients should be closely monitored.[30] The Neoadjuvant Treatment for Advanced Rectal Carcinoma trial (NACRE), is currently enrolling patients ≥75 years, comparing SCRT *vs.* nCRT in terms of efficacy and treatment-related morbidity (NCT02551237). Longer intervals may increase clinical tumour response rates and are an option if an organ preservation approach is sought.[31]

Local excision for early rectal cancer

One-third of screen detected rectal cancers are endoscopic retrograde cholangiography (ERC) endoluminal yet >90% undergo TME.[32] Minimally invasive endoscopic and transanal surgical techniques have been developed to allow for less invasive resection of ERC.[33] LE is deemed to be appropriate for management with curative intent of some ERC.[34] In appropriately selected patients, LE may provide a less risky alternative to TME and confer a number of benefits, including organ preservation, improved functional outcomes, decreased overall morbidity, operating time, and length of in-hospital stay.[35] This is particularly relevant to frail comorbid patients unable to undergo TME.

Morbidity and mortality

Overall mortality with LE is low (0–3%), and morbidity ranges from 10 to 45%. The most common risk is bleeding, with infection being a rarer occurrence.[36,37] Overall morbidity increases with patient age; approximately 20% in <75 years, 25% in those aged 75–84 and 35% in those aged >85 years.[25] Elderly patients are more likely to require surgical intervention when an adverse outcome occurs.[25]

The 'watch and wait' approach

Elderly patients with a cCR on clinical and radiological re-evaluation may be offered a W&W approach.[38] Many patients chose the W&W strategy in order to avoid a permanent stoma or the long-term functional problems associated with TME surgery.[38] Haak et al. specifically assessed the role of W&W in 43 elderly patients. Outcomes in this study were promising, with a three-year local regrowth-free rate of 88% and a three-year non-regrowth disease-free survival of 91%. Overall survival was 97% with a three-year colostomy-free survival of 93%. Safety of this approach was achieved in this group with no major impact on functional outcomes.[39]

In addition to the goal of increasing the QoL in operable patients, there is the additional benefit of avoiding major surgery in frail elderly patients with substantial comorbidities. Smith et al. used a model to compare three cohorts of men: 60-year-olds with mild comorbidities, 80-year-olds with minor comorbidities, and 80-year-olds with significant comorbidities. Patients with a cCR after nCRT were followed by a W&W protocol or radical surgery. Absolute survival was similar in the 60-year-old cohort. However, in both fit 80-year-olds and those with comorbidities, there was a 10.1% survival advantage at one year in those who underwent a W&W approach. There were no differences between groups in disease-free survival (DFS) or quality-adjusted life years (QALY). This model suggests elderly patients may have the most to gain from W&W after cCR.[40]

LE following neoadjuvant therapy

In contrast to locally advanced rectal cancer (LARC), currently neoadjuvant therapy is not routinely indicated for ERC and approximately one-quarter of all TME operations performed in the UK are for non-irradiated pT1/T2 ERC.[41] One proposed experimental strategy to overcome this is radiotherapy to treat microscopic mesorectal lymph node metastasis (LNM) and contribute to tumour downsizing prior to LE.[42] Patients with clinically staged cT1 and cT2 rectal cancers, have very high rates of pCR after nCRT in the region of 30–40%[43] and as such, this strategy could be considered in older or more frail patients not considered fit enough for major resection. However, it is important to consider that multiple treatments can give rise to cumulative toxicities that detract from the benefits of organ preservation, particularly in older patients or frail patients.[42,44]

A small randomized trial was the first to suggest that LE after nCRT was safe compared to TME in cT2 tumours less than 3 cm in size.[45] This was subsequently seen in the CARTS[46] and ACOSOG Z6041 study.[44] The CARTS study demonstrated organ preservation was achievable in two-thirds of patients with good long-term outcomes, while the ACOSOG Z6041 demonstrated a low three-year LR rate. GRECCAR 2 demonstrated that long-term oncological outcomes in organ preservation are comparable to TME, suggesting that patients with cT2/T3 tumours demonstrating a good clinical response can be treated by LE.[42]

An alternative to combination nCRT with reduced toxicity is SCRT. The efficacy of SCRT compared with nCRT for prevention of LR is supported by two phase 3 trials, with SCRT showing reduced toxicity.[28,29] Similarly, SCRT with delayed LE may provide safe and effective primary organ preservation for frail patient[47]; however, excessive surgical morbidity has also been reported.[48] The TREC study, the first randomized controlled trial (RCT) to assign patients with ERC to organ preservation (via short-SCRT and delayed LE) or upfront radical surgery (TME), has published its results.[49] It also reported on patients for whom randomization was considered inappropriate due to clinical indication. Non-randomized patients who underwent organ preservation were older than randomized patients and more likely to have life-limiting comorbidities. Interestingly, 81% of eligible patients approached for TREC took part and 36% were randomly assigned, highlighting the acceptability of an organ preservation approach if it is offered and the feasibility of randomly assigning patients to substantially different treatment approaches.[49] Overall, SCRT followed by LE achieved high levels of organ preservation in both the randomized (70%) and non-randomized (92%) cohorts, with relatively low morbidity and indications of improved quality of life.[49]

Local excision in the palliative setting

LE has gained popularity in recent years for early rectal tumours without unfavourable oncologic prognostic factors.[50] It has however been employed also in the palliative setting and remains in use today. Untreated LARC or locally recurrent rectal cancer may lead to obstruction or symptoms such as intractable pain and bleeding, causing significant distress for patients and consequences for functional status.[51] While the immediate treatment of an obstructing tumour typically consists of resection, defunctioning stoma, or self-expanding metallic stent where feasible,[52] this approach may not be as effective in relieving additional symptoms such as pain and bleeding.[53] Where selected appropriately, LE can offer this cohort relief with decreased morbidity and recovery time compared to that of formal resection[54] and avoidance of a stoma.

For unresectable stage IV disease requiring palliative intervention, Chen et al.[55] compared transanal endoscopic LE to open resection. Their results highlighted significantly lower morbidity in the LE group ($p = 0.049$) and a trend towards decreased stoma formation (17% vs. 28% in open). The patient should be counselled on the suboptimal oncologic nature of this procedure as a palliative approach and aware that local recurrence rates remain as high as 58% and 79% in T3 and T4 tumours.[56,57] Furthermore, the muscle wall and mesorectum left intact following local resection may harbour residual tumour.

Chemotherapy in the palliative setting

Systemic chemotherapy may be utilized as an organ-preserving strategy and improve overall survival in the asymptomatic patient undergoing treatment with palliative intent.[58] It may be utilized either in isolation or as an adjunct to LE and/or radiotherapy in the palliative setting. Historically, there was a move towards prophylactic formal resection within this group due to concern that the primary tumour would become symptomatic with disease progression. Studies have demonstrated, however, that asymptomatic patients are more likely to die from their disease prior to the onset of symptoms pertaining to the primary tumour.[52] Furthermore, the morbidity and mortality in patients with asymptomatic stage IV disease who undergo surgery appear to be unjustifiably high when compared to the rate of asymptomatic patients treated non-operatively in the first instance who ultimately require surgical intervention.[59]

The addition of oxaliplatin and irinotecan in recent years to the more traditional regimen of fluorouracil (FU) and leucovorin confers improved survival.[60,61] The GERCOR study[58] demonstrated median overall survival of 21.5 months in patients treated initially with FOLFIRI (leucovorin, fluorouracil, irinotecan) and FOLFOX (leucovorin, fluorouracil, oxaliplatin) as second-line versus 20.6 months for FOLFOX followed by FOLFIRI. This compares favourably to overall survival data from prior studies examining both FU and leucovorin alone or in conjunction with irinotecan or oxaliplatin.[62,63]

Radiotherapy in the palliative setting

Symptom control and quality of life are the ultimate goals of any palliative intervention for rectal cancer. Palliative radiotherapy can be utilized to achieve these but is reportedly underused.[64] Cameron et al.[65] conducted a systematic review of the efficacy and toxicity of palliative external beam radiotherapy across 27 publications. Between 56% and 100% of patients had a good symptomatic response. Toxicity was inconsistently reported, however, mild to moderate toxicity was the most severe level observed within patient cohorts. A more recent prospective multicentre study by Cameron et al.[66] demonstrated improved or complete resolution of symptoms (pain, bleeding, and rectal dysfunction) in 60% of patients (28/47) following a course of radiotherapy consisting of a median total dose of 36 Gy delivered in 3 Gy fraction sizes. Symptoms of radiation toxicity reported were low-grade (1–2) and transient in most cases.

With regards to dosage, the systematic review by Cameron et al.[65] reported total doses most frequently between 30 and 60 Gy with a daily fraction size of 2 Gy most commonly. There has been a trend towards 'hypofractionated treatment' in more recent times however, the rationale being that minimal time is spent by patients in hospital. This comprises a higher dosage of radiation at each attendance rather than the more conventional approach of smaller daily fraction sizes of up to 2.0 Gy. While hypofractionated treatments may be associated with an increased risk of late toxicity, the risk of this in a palliative patient with a reduced life expectancy may be offset by the more immediate benefits.[67] This must be tailored on an individual basis however and emphasizes the importance of appropriate patient selection for this approach.

References

1. Siegel RL, Miller KD, Goding Sauer A, et al. Colorectal cancer statistics, 2020. *CA Cancer J Clin*. 2020;70(3):145–64.
2. Feng MA, McMillan DT, Crowell K, Muss H, Nielsen ME, Smith AB. Geriatric assessment in surgical oncology: a systematic review. *J Surg Res*. 2015;193(1):265–72.
3. Montroni I, Ugolini G, Saur NM, et al. Personalized management of elderly patients with rectal cancer: Expert recommendations of the European Society of Surgical Oncology, European Society of Coloproctology, International Society of Geriatric Oncology, and American College of Surgeons Commission on Cancer. *Eur J Surg Oncol*. 2018;44(11):1685–702.
4. De Angelis R, Sant M, Coleman MP, et al. Cancer survival in Europe 1999–2007 by country and age: results of EUROCARE-5—a population-based study. *Lancet Oncol*. 2014;15(1):23–4.
5. Kessler H, Hermanek P, Jr., Wiebelt H. Operative mortality in carcinoma of the rectum. Results of the German Multicentre Study. *Int J Colorectal Dis*. 1993;8(3):158–66.
6. Puig-La Calle J, Quayle J, Thaler H, et al. Favorable short-term and long-term outcome after elective radical rectal cancer resection in patients 75 years of age or older. *Dis Colon Rectum*. 2000;43(12):1704–9.
7. Rutten HJ, den Dulk M, Lemmens VE, van de Velde CJ, Marijnen CA. Controversies of total mesorectal excision for rectal cancer in elderly patients. *Lancet Oncol*. 2008;9(5):494–501.
8. NCIN. Major resections by cancer site, in England; 2006 to 2010. National Cancer Intelligence Network short report. Stage Breakdown by CCG 2014. London: NCIN. 2016: 1–10. http://www.ncin.org.uk/about_ncin/major_resections.
9. Lawler M, Alsina D, Adams RA, et al. Critical research gaps and recommendations to inform research prioritisation for more effective prevention and improved outcomes in colorectal cancer. *Gut*. 2018;67(1):179–93.
10. Bufalari A, Giustozzi G, Burattini MF, et al. Rectal cancer surgery in the elderly: a multivariate analysis of outcome risk factors. *J Surg Oncol*. 2006;93(3):173–80.
11. Partridge JS, Harari D, Dhesi JK. Frailty in the older surgical patient: a review. *Age Ageing*. 2012;41(2):142–7.
12. Montroni I, Ugolini G, Saur NM, et al. Personalized management of elderly patients with rectal cancer: expert recommendations of the European Society of Surgical Oncology, European Society of Coloproctology, International Society of Geriatric Oncology, and American College of Surgeons Commission on Cancer. *Eur J Surg Oncol*. 2018;44(11):1685–702.
13. Bruns ER, van den Heuvel B, Buskens CJ, et al. The effects of physical prehabilitation in elderly patients undergoing colorectal surgery: a systematic review. *Colorectal Dis*. 2016;18(8):267–77.
14. Samuelsson KS, Egenvall M, Klarin I, Lökk J, Gunnarsson U. Preoperative geriatric assessment and follow-up of patients older than 75 years undergoing elective surgery for suspected colorectal cancer. *J Geriatr Oncol*. 2019;10(5):709–15.

15. Huisman MG, Van Leeuwen BL, Ugolini G, et al. 'Timed Up & Go': a screening tool for predicting 30-day morbidity in onco-geriatric surgical patients? A multicenter cohort study. *PloS One*. 2014;9(1):e86863.
16. Kristjansson SR, Nesbakken A, Jordhøy MS, et al. Comprehensive geriatric assessment can predict complications in elderly patients after elective surgery for colorectal cancer: a prospective observational cohort study. *Crit Rev Oncol Hematol*. 2010;76(3):208–17.
17. Li C, Carli F, Lee L, et al. Impact of a trimodal prehabilitation program on functional recovery after colorectal cancer surgery: a pilot study. *Surg Endosc*. 2013;27(4):1072–82.
18. Minnella EM, Awasthi R, Gillis C, et al. Patients with poor baseline walking capacity are most likely to improve their functional status with multimodal prehabilitation. *Surgery*. 2016;160(4):1070–9.
19. van Rooijen SJ, Molenaar CJL, Schep G, et al. Making patients fit for surgery: introducing a four pillar multimodal prehabilitation program in colorectal cancer. *Am J Phys Med Rehabil*. Oct;98(10):888–96.
20. Burden ST, Hill J, Shaffer JL, Todd C. Nutritional status of preoperative colorectal cancer patients. *J Hum Nutr Diet*. 2010;23(4):402–7.
21. Huisman M, Veronese G, Audisio R, et al. Poor nutritional status is associated with other geriatric domain impairments and adverse postoperative outcomes in onco-geriatric surgical patients—a multicentre cohort study. *Eur J Surg Oncol (EJSO)*. 2016;42(7):1009–17.
22. Gillis C, Loiselle S-E, Fiore Jr JF, et al. Prehabilitation with whey protein supplementation on perioperative functional exercise capacity in patients undergoing colorectal resection for cancer: a pilot double-blinded randomized placebo-controlled trial. *J Acad Nutr Dietetics*. 2016;116(5):802–12.
23. Lemmens VE, Janssen-Heijnen ML, Houterman S, et al. Which comorbid conditions predict complications after surgery for colorectal cancer? *World J Surg*. 2007;31(1):192–9.
24. Erichsen R, Horvath-Puho E, Iversen L, Lash T, Sørensen HT. Does comorbidity interact with colorectal cancer to increase mortality? A nationwide population-based cohort study. *Br J Cancer*. 2013;109(7):2005.
25. Sevak S, Gregoir T, Wolthuis A, Albert M. How can we utilize local excision to help, not harm, geriatric patients with rectal cancer? *Eur J Surg Oncol*. 2020;46(3):344–8.
26. Janssen-Heijnen ML, Maas HA, Houterman S, Lemmens VE, Rutten HJ, Coebergh JW. Comorbidity in older surgical cancer patients: influence on patient care and outcome. *Eur J Cancer*. 2007;43(15):2179–93.
27. De Marco MF, Janssen-Heijnen ML, van der Heijden LH, Coebergh JW. Comorbidity and colorectal cancer according to subsite and stage: a population-based study. *Eur J Cancer*. 2000;36(1):95–9.
28. Ngan SY, Burmeister B, Fisher RJ, et al. Randomized trial of short-course radiotherapy versus long-course chemoradiation comparing rates of local recurrence in patients with T3 rectal cancer: Trans-Tasman Radiation Oncology Group trial 01.04. *J Clin Oncol*. 2012;30(31):3827–33.
29. Bujko K, Nowacki MP, Nasierowska-Guttmejer A, Michalski W, Bebenek M, Kryj M. Long-term results of a randomized trial comparing preoperative short-course radiotherapy with preoperative conventionally fractionated chemoradiation for rectal cancer. *Br J Surg*. 2006;93(10):1215–23.
30. Bahadoer RR, Dijkstra EA, van Etten B, et al. Short-course radiotherapy followed by chemotherapy before total mesorectal excision (TME) versus preoperative chemoradiotherapy, TME, and optional adjuvant chemotherapy in locally advanced rectal cancer (RAPIDO): a randomised, open-label, phase 3 trial. *Lancet Oncol*. 2021;22(1):29–42.

31. Ryan EJ, O'Sullivan DP, Kelly ME, et al. Meta-analysis of the effect of extending the interval after long-course chemoradiotherapy before surgery in locally advanced rectal cancer. *Br J Surg.* 2019;106(10):1298–310.
32. National Bowel Cancer Audit Project Team. National Bowel Cancer Audit Report 2015. London: Health and Social Care Information Centre, 2015. https://digital.nhs.uk/data-and-information/publications/statistical/national-bowel-cancer-audit/national-bowel-cancer-audit-report-2015.
33. Naughton AP, Ryan É J, Bardon CT, et al. Endoscopic management versus transanal surgery for early primary or early locally recurrent rectal neoplasms-a systematic review and meta-analysis. *Int J Colorectal Dis.* 2020;35(12):2347–59.
34. Glynne-Jones R, Wyrwicz L, Tiret E, et al. Rectal cancer: ESMO Clinical Practice Guidelines for diagnosis, treatment and follow-up. *Ann Oncol.* 2017;28(suppl_4):iv22–iv40.
35. Peeters KC, Marijnen CA, Nagtegaal ID, et al. The TME trial after a median follow-up of 6 years: increased local control but no survival benefit in irradiated patients with resectable rectal carcinoma. *Ann Surg.* 2007;246(5):693–701.
36. Bach S, Hill J, Monson J, et al. Association of coloproctology of Great Britain and Ireland Transanal Endoscopic Microsurgery (TEM) Collaboration. A predictive model for local recurrence after transanal endoscopic microsurgery for rectal cancer. *Br J Surg.* 2009;96(3):280–90.
37. Marks JH, Valsdottir E, DeNittis A, et al. Transanal endoscopic microsurgery for the treatment of rectal cancer: comparison of wound complication rates with and without neoadjuvant radiation therapy. *Surg Endosc.* 2009;23(5):1081–7.
38. Beets GL, Figueiredo NL, Habr-Gama A, van de Velde CJ. A new paradigm for rectal cancer: organ preservation: introducing the International Watch & Wait Database (IWWD). *Eur J Surg Oncol.* 2015;41(12):1562–4.
39. Haak HE, Maas M, Lambregts DMJ, Beets-Tan RGH, Beets GL. Is watch and wait a safe and effective way to treat rectal cancer in older patients? *Eur J Surg Oncol.* 2020;46(3):358–62.
40. Smith FM, Rao C, Perez RO, et al. Avoiding radical surgery improves early survival in elderly patients with rectal cancer, demonstrating complete clinical response after neoadjuvant therapy: results of a decision-analytic model. *Dis Colon Rectum.* 2015;58(2):159–71.
41. Boyle J, Braun M, Hill J, et al. National Bowel Cancer Audit: annual report 2018. December, 2018. https://www.nboca.org.uk/content/uploads/2018/12/NBOCA-annual-report2018.pdf.
42. Rullier E, Vendrely V, Asselineau J, et al. Organ preservation with chemoradiotherapy plus local excision for rectal cancer: 5-year results of the GRECCAR 2 randomised trial. *Lancet Gastroenterol Hepatol.* 2020;5(5):465–74.
43. Maas M, Nelemans PJ, Valentini V, et al. Long-term outcome in patients with a pathological complete response after chemoradiation for rectal cancer: a pooled analysis of individual patient data. *Lancet Oncol.* 2010;11(9):835–44.
44. Garcia-Aguilar J, Renfro LA, Chow OS, et al. Organ preservation for clinical T2N0 distal rectal cancer using neoadjuvant chemoradiotherapy and local excision (ACOSOG Z6041): results of an open-label, single-arm, multi-institutional, phase 2 trial. *Lancet Oncol.* 2015;16(15):1537–46.
45. Lezoche E, Baldarelli M, Lezoche G, Paganini A, Gesuita R, Guerrieri M. Randomized clinical trial of endoluminal locoregional resection versus laparoscopic total mesorectal excision for T2 rectal cancer after neoadjuvant therapy. *Br J Surg.* 2012;99(9):1211–18.
46. Verseveld M, De Graaf E, Verhoef C, et al. Chemoradiation therapy for rectal cancer in the distal rectum followed by organ-sparing transanal endoscopic microsurgery (CARTS study). *Br J Surg.* 2015;102(7):853–60.

47. Smart CJ, Korsgen S, Hill J, et al. Multicentre study of short-course radiotherapy and transanal endoscopic microsurgery for early rectal cancer. *Br J Surg.* 2016;103(8):1069–75.
48. Arezzo A, Arolfo S, Allaix ME, et al. Results of neoadjuvant short-course radiation therapy followed by transanal endoscopic microsurgery for T1-T2 N0 extraperitoneal rectal cancer. Article. *Int J Radiat Oncol Biol Phys.* 2015;92(2):299–306.
49. Bach SP, Gilbert A, Brock K, et al. Radical surgery versus organ preservation via short-course radiotherapy followed by transanal endoscopic microsurgery for early-stage rectal cancer (TREC): a randomised, open-label feasibility study. *Lancet Gastroenterol Hepatol.* 2021;6(2):92–105.
50. Beaton C, Twine C, Williams G, Radcliffe A. Systematic review and meta-analysis of histopathological factors influencing the risk of lymph node metastasis in early colorectal cancer. *Colorectal Dis.* 2013;15(7):788–97.
51. Heriot K. Rectal cancer recurrence: factors and mechanisms. *Colorectal Dis.* 2000;2(3):126–36.
52. Wasserberg N, Kaufman HS. Palliation of colorectal cancer. *Surg Oncol.* 2007;16(4):299–310.
53. Türler A, Schäfer H, Pichlmaier H. Role of transanal endoscopic microsurgery in the palliative treatment of rectal cancer. *Scand J Gastroenterol.* 1997;32(1):58–61.
54. You YN, Baxter NN, Stewart A, Nelson H. Is the increasing rate of local excision for stage I rectal cancer in the United States justified?: a nationwide cohort study from the National Cancer Database. *Ann Surg.* 2007;245(5):726.
55. Chen H, George BD, Kaufian HS, Malaki MB, Mortensen NJM, Kett Lewell MG. Endoscopic transanal resection provides palliation equivalent to transabdominal resection in patients with metastatic rectal cancer. *J Gastrointest Surg.* 2001;5(3):282–6.
56. Mellgren A, Sirivongs P, Rothenberger DA, Madoff RD, García-Aguilar J. Is local excision adequate therapy for early rectal cancer? *Dis Colon Rectum.* 2000;43(8):1064–71.
57. den Dekker N, Van Oostendorp SE, Tuynman JB. Organ preservation and palliative options for rectal cancer. In: Atallah, S., ed. Transanal Minimally Invasive Surgery (TAMIS) and Transanal Total Mesorectal Excision (taTME). Cham, Switzerland: Springer; 2019:49–55.
58. Tournigand C, André T, Achille E, et al. FOLFIRI followed by FOLFOX6 or the reverse sequence in advanced colorectal cancer: a randomized GERCOR study. *J Clin Oncol.* 2004;22(2):229–37.
59. Scoggins CR, Meszoely IM, Blanke CD, Beauchamp RD, Leach SD. Nonoperative management of primary colorectal cancer in patients with stage IV disease. *Ann Surg Oncol.* 1999;6(7):651–7.
60. Cunningham D, Pyrhönen S, James RD, et al. Randomised trial of irinotecan plus supportive care versus supportive care alone after fluorouracil failure for patients with metastatic colorectal cancer. *Lancet.* 1998;352(9138):1413–18.
61. Douillard J, Cunningham D, Roth A, et al. Irinotecan combined with fluorouracil compared with fluorouracil alone as first-line treatment for metastatic colorectal cancer: a multicentre randomised trial. *Lancet.* 2000;355(9209):1041–7.
62. Saltz LB, Cox JV, Blanke C, et al. Irinotecan plus fluorouracil and leucovorin for metastatic colorectal cancer. *N Engl J Med.* 2000;343(13):905–14.
63. Jonker D, Rumble RB, Maroun J, Care GCDSGCCOsPiE-B. Role of oxaliplatin combined with 5-fluorouracil and folinic acid in the first-and second-line treatment of advanced colorectal cancer. *Curr Oncol.* 2006;13(5):173.
64. Delaney G, Jacob S, Featherstone C, Barton M. The role of radiotherapy in cancer treatment: estimating optimal utilization from a review of evidence-based clinical guidelines. *Cancer.* 2005;104(6):1129–37.

65. Cameron MG, Kersten C, Vistad I, Fosså S, Guren MG. Palliative pelvic radiotherapy of symptomatic incurable rectal cancer—a systematic review. *Acta Oncologica.* 2014;53(2):164–73.
66. Cameron MG, Kersten C, Vistad I, et al. Palliative pelvic radiotherapy for symptomatic rectal cancer–a prospective multicenter study. *Acta Oncologica*. 2016;55(12):1400–7.
67. Lutz ST, Jones J, Chow E. Role of radiation therapy in palliative care of the patient with cancer. *J Clin Oncol.* 2014;32(26):2913.

13
Quality of life after organ preservation for rectal cancer

Jesse Fischer, Andrew McCombie, and Frank A. Frizelle

Introduction

When examining QoL there are several questions that need to be considered, and as such alter how one interprets the published studies.

1. What is QoL and how and when do we best measure it in these patients so as to accurately reflect the components of care that are altered in the different treatment paradigms?
2. What is the relevant patient population to study, is it just patients who have successful OP, or should it be those who start down the path of OP with CRT irrespective of whether successfully treated with OP or undergo TME?

What is quality of life and how and when do we best measure it in these patients so as to accurately reflect the components of care that are altered in the different treatment paradigms?

What is quality of life?

QoL is defined as a person's self-evaluation of their present level of functioning in day-to-day living and satisfaction with it as compared to what they perceive to be optimal.[1] QoL is subjective, multidimensional, dynamic, and patient-centred, and comprises physical, functional, emotional, and social well-being domains.[2] In the context of oncology, it is easy to see how these domains can be affected: cancer patients can experience pain and nausea (i.e. physical), impaired ability to carry out one's role at home or work (i.e. functional), depression and anguish (i.e. emotional), and difficulty maintaining relationships with family and friends (i.e. social). In the rectal cancer treatment context, the important aspects reflect bowel, urological, and sexual function to a greater degree than in other contexts.

Why is QoL important?

QoL is growing in importance in clinical practice as survival improves.[3] Society is recognizing the importance of quality as distinct from quantity of life. The increasing recognition of the importance of QoL is seen in society publicly debating such issues as euthanasia.

How do we assess QoL?

Due to the subjective nature of QoL, there are numerous ways of measuring it. One method of measuring QoL is asking the individual what they believe to be the most important components of their own QoL and rating them themselves.[4] This method, while no doubt frustrating for those who prefer a more objective and clear-cut method, has the great advantage of not making the speculative assumption that all people have the same internal standards, values, and conceptualization of QoL.

When the subjective and hybrid approach to measuring QoL is not desired, generic or disease-specific (cancer-specific or even colorectal-cancer-specific) instruments can be used.[5] Both these types of instruments assume that all aspects of QoL are equally important to all people. Generic instruments, such as the EQ-5D-5L[6] or SF-12,[7] are useful for comparing individuals to the general population or people without cancer, whereas disease-specific instruments, such as QLQ-CR29[8] and FACT-C,[9] are more sensitive to aspects specific to malignancy (e.g. bowel-related symptoms) and changes within a patient over time.

QoL assessment is also considered with length of survival with the use of quality-adjusted life years (QALYs). QALYs measure quality multiplied by length of survival with the EQ-5D-5L being commonly used for this. Clinical and health economic decision-making is increasingly aiming to maximize QALYs as opposed to quality or survival alone.[10]

The different tools to assess QoL therefore can produce heterogeneous results from the same study population and therefore comparing results between studies which use different methods can be difficult.

Response shift

Response shift occurs when a patient self-reports different QoL over time, even when it would seem their QoL has not changed to the outside observer (or a patient reports no change in QoL when it would seem the QoL has changed to the outside observer).[11] In response shift, the patient recalibrates their internal standards and definition of what constitutes a 'good' QoL for them when they are faced with a serious illness.[12] Response shift results from a change in the meaning of one's self-assessment of QoL due to a change in the person's (1) internal standards of measurement (i.e. recalibration), (2) values (i.e. reprioritization), and/or (3) definition of QoL (i.e. reconceptualization). This means that a patient's QoL score can return to pretreatment levels, but in reality their QoL can appear different to an outside observer, and they have adapted psychologically to changes in their body.

Who is the relevant patient population?

The issue here is that two or three groups of distinctly different patients are included in studies examining QoL after OP.

- Group (1): those with locally advanced rectal cancer who would receive preoperative chemoradiation as standard treatment.
- Group (2): those with early rectal cancer who only receive chemoradiation as part of an OP pathway.

In this second group, all patients receive preoperative chemoradiation when otherwise they would have gone straight to surgery, and therefore group 2 can be divided into two subgroups:

- Group 2a (the minority, 15–35%): those who achieve a clinical complete response on the OP pathway.
- Group 2b (the majority): those who don't achieve a clinical complete response and progress to TME.

Both 2a and 2b are exposed to the short-term and long-term effects of preoperative chemoradiation.

If we assume the intention-to-treat paradigm as we do with most studies, then all patients in group 2 must be considered the treatment group. For group 1 it is more debatable who the study population is as all patients would be considered for preoperative CRT as standard treatment.

When do we measure quality of life?

When we measure QoL affects the outcome of the assessment. Radiation causes a progressive obliterative end arteritis and as such the microscopic ischaemic damage and functional impact is progressive over time. As a result function and therefore QoL might deteriorate with time. Physiological implications include nerve dysfunction, loss of rectal compliance, and direct damage to the anal sphincter complex. The longer we wait the more response shift become important, and patients QoL improves.

Effects of pelvic radiation on functional outcome

Studies from the 1990s uncovered that patients who had preoperative chemoradiation had a worse functional outcome than those who went direct to surgery, however QoL itself was not directly measured.

Kollmorgen et al.[13] demonstrated that for carefully selected patient groups the group that had postoperative chemoradiotherapy had more bowel movements per day than the group that did not have radiation therapy (median 7 vs. median 2, p <0.001); the former group had 'clustering' of bowel movements more often (42% vs. 3%, p <0.001), had nighttime movements more often (46% vs. 14%, p <0.001), had occasional or frequent incontinence more often (39% and 17% vs. 7% and 0%, p <0.001), wore a pad more often (41% vs. 10%, p <0.001), and were unable to defer defecation for more than 15 minutes more often (78% vs. 19%, p <0.001). The group that had chemoradiotherapy also had stool of liquid consistency, used antidiarrheal medications, had perianal skin irritation, were unable to differentiate stool from gas, and needed to defecate again within 30 minutes of a movement significantly more often than the group that did not receive chemoradiotherapy.

The data on preoperative chemoradiotherapy is similar to postoperative chemoradiotherapy. Patients who receive neoadjuvant treatment and undergo anterior resection for distal rectal tumours are at risk of developing low anterior resection syndrome (LARS), which can present with a myriad of symptoms including faecal incontinence, faecal urgency, and abdominal bloating. The prevalence of LARS was found to be up to 42% of patients having a low anterior resection.[14] The pathophysiology of this syndrome is attributed to impaired function of the anal sphincters, colonic dysmotility, and dysfunction of the neorectal reservoir.[14] While reconstructive techniques did alter the extent that LARS affected patients,[15,16] the use of radiation had the most dramatic effect.[14]

Neural factors however also play a significant role in the development of LARS. Neural dysfunction can occur post-treatment either as a result of denervation post-surgery or as a consequence of radiotherapy. In a cross-sectional study on rectal cancer patients published in 2013, 41% of the total patient cohort of 938 experienced LARS.[17] The authors observed that those who received neoadjuvant radiotherapy (long or short course) and TME surgery had an increased risk of developing LARS.

In a 14-year follow-up study of patients enrolled in the Dutch Rectal Cancer Trial, the authors observed a 46% incidence of LARS in the 242 patients who responded to questionnaires.[18] Neoadjuvant radiotherapy and age <75 years were found to be significant risk factors. Furthermore, LARS was also associated with a reduction in Health-Related Quality of Life (HRQOL). A recent study by Kupsch et al.[19,20] reported a significant reduction in HRQOL scores for patients reporting major LARS using the standardized EORCT-30 and CR38 questionnaire. Patients with major LARS scored 56 ± 19 compared to minor/no LARS who scored 67 ± 20 (p <0.001).

These studies demonstrate that long-term effects of CRT do affect function, and impacts on assessments of QoL, in patients who have also had a rectal resection. The issue is the balance between those who receive CRT for early rectal cancer as part of an OP pathway but fail to achieve OP and subsequently undergo TME, against those who avoid surgery following successful OP, and then the third group of those who have just surgery and no CRT. The analysis of QoL between these groups across the whole population of those with localized rectal cancer is difficult.

Quality of life after organ preservation

Most of the studies on OP have focused on oncological outcome examining aspects such as overall and cancer-free survival, patterns of treatment failure, and local recurrence. The limited number of studies on QoL have often been spin-off studies from these oncological outcome studies. The results are summarized in Table 13.1.

In the study by Habr-Gama et al.[21] consecutive patients with early stage localized distal rectal cancer underwent neoadjuvant chemoradiation (50.4–54 Gy and 5-fluorouracil-based chemotherapy). Patients with a clinically complete response were managed by watch-and-wait. Patients with near-complete response (≤3 cm, ycT1-2N0) were managed by transanal endoscopic microsurgery (TEM). Functional outcomes were determined by anorectal manometry, Faecal Incontinence Index, and QoL assessment. Baseline features were similar between groups. Patients undergoing TEM had worse resting/squeeze pressures ($p = 0.004$) and rectal capacity ($p = 0.002$). In addition, their incontinence scores (2.3 vs. 6.5; $p < 0.001$) and QoL questionnaire responses (in all domains; $p \leq 0.01$) were significantly worse in comparison with patients undergoing watch-and-wait.

The study from a Maastricht group by Hupkins et al.[22] examined the QoL of watch-and-wait patients with a matched-controlled group of patients who underwent chemoradiation and surgery (total mesorectal excision group). The study population consisted of two groups: 41 patients after a watch-and-wait policy and 41 matched patients after chemoradiation and surgery. Patients were matched on sex, age, tumour stage, and tumour height, and all patients had a minimum follow-up of 2 years. The study showed that the watch-and-wait group showed better physical and cognitive function, better physical and emotional roles, and better global health status compared with the total mesorectal excision group. The watch-and-wait patients showed fewer problems with defecation and sexual and urinary tract function. This was a good quality study; however, it only focused on watch-and-wait patients who achieved a sustained complete response for two years, and patients who had local failure and subsequent resection were excluded.

The US-based study from Memorial Sloan Kettering and the Mayo Clinic[23] was a prospective study that assessed anorectal function and QoL of patients with T2N0 rectal cancer who were treated with an alternative approach. Anorectal function and QoL were assessed at enrolment and one year postoperatively with the Faecal Incontinence Severity Index, Faecal Incontinence Quality of Life scale, and Functional Assessment of Cancer Therapy-Colorectal Questionnaire. Seventy-one patients (98%) were evaluated at enrolment and 66 (92%) at 1 year. Compared with baseline, no significant differences were found on Faecal Incontinence Severity Index scores at 1 year. Faecal Incontinence QoL results were significantly worse in the lifestyle ($p < 0.001$), coping/behaviour ($p < 0.001$), and embarrassment ($p = 0.002$) domains. There were no differences in the Functional Assessment of Cancer Therapy overall score, but the physical well-being subscale was significantly worse and emotional

Table 13.1 Quality of life study results

First author (year)	Study design	Target group/ Comparison	Outcome measure(s)	Results	Follow-up
Habr-Gama (2016)	Prospective cohort study	cCR treated with W&W (n = 53) vs. near-cCR treated with TEM (n = 29). Total n = 82	Anorectal manometry, CCII, FIQL	TEM patients generally had worse function than W&W patients including lower anorectal manometry pressures and rectal capacity, higher CCII scores (6.5 vs. 2.3 [p <0.001]), worse FIQL across lifestyle, coping/behaviour, depression/self-perception and embarrassment domains	Median 35.7 months
Hupkens (2017)	Matched-controlled study	W&W (n = 41) vs. nCRT and TME (n = 41). Total n s = 82	SF-36, EORTC-QLQ-CR38, EORTC-QLQCR30, Vaizey incontinence score, LARS score, IIEF, FSFI, IPSS	OP patients reported better QoL across multiple domains of SF-36 (physical function, physical role and emotional role) but TME reported better general health. OP patients reported better function across multiple domains of EORTC-QLQ-C30 (physical functioning, role functioning, cognitive functioning), and EORTC-QLQ-C38 (better body image and better QoL in last week). TME reported more FI than W&W on LARS and Vaizey scores. No difference in sexual function on FSFI and IIEF but EORTC-QLQ-CR38 showed better sexual function in W&W patients. IPSS reported less urinary dysfunction in W&W group	2 years minimum
Lynn (2017)	Prospective assessment within a multicentre phase 2 trial	cT2N0 treated with nCRT and local excision. Total n = sss71	FISI, FIQL, FACT-C	Compared with baseline, there was no difference in FISI or FACT-C overall but several domains of FIQL were impaired (lifestyle coping/behaviour and embarrassment)	1 year minimum
Martens (2016)	Prospective cohort study	cCR treated with W&W (n = 22) vs. near-cCR treated with TEM (n = 7). Total n = 29	Vaizey incontinence score	One OP patient had major incontinence compared with three TEM patients. Mean total Vaizey score of W&W patients was 3.4 (SD = 3.9), indicating good continence, compared with 9.7 (SD = 5.1) in TEM patients (p =*.003*)	3 years minimum
van der Sande (2019)	Cross-sectional study	W&W patients. Total n = 33	Anorectal manometry, Vaizey incontinence score, LARS score	Mean anal resting pressure 30 +/− 12 mmHg and mean anal squeeze pressure 104 +/− 41 mmHg. Mean LARS score 23.4 +/ − 11.3 (33.3% of patients had major LARS) and mean Vaizey score 4.3 +/− 4.1	2 years minimum (median 38 months)

well-being was improved after surgery. Treatment with the original chemoradiation regimen predicted worse depression/self-perception and embarrassment scores in the Faecal Incontinence QoL, and male sex was predictive of worse scores in the Functional Assessment of Cancer Therapy overall score and trial outcome index. Despite being a well-designed prospective study it is has a small sample size, and relatively short follow-up.

Another study by the Maastricht group authors reported by Martens et al.[24] examined patients where organ preservation was offered. Watch-and-wait was offered after a cCR, and two options were offered for near-cCR: TEM or reassessment after three months. Functional outcome was assessed with colostomy-free survival and Vaizey incontinence score (0 = perfect continence, 24 = totally incontinent). One hundred patients were included, with median follow-up of 41.1 months. Sixty-one had cCR at initial response assessment. Thirty-nine had near-cCR, of whom 24 developed cCR at the second assessment and 15 patients underwent TEM (9 ypT0, 1 ypT1, 5 ypT2). Fifteen patients developed a local regrowth (12 luminal, 3 nodal), all were salvageable, and occurred within 25 months. Colostomy-free survival was 94.8% (95% CI = 88.0% to 97.8%). Despite the initial large numbers only 29 patients completed the questionnaires, of which 22 were in the watch-and-wait arm and seven had undergone after TEM excision. This showed good continence after watch-and-wait (Vaizey = 3.4, SD = 3.9) and moderate after TEM (Vaizey = 9.7, SD = 5.1). Patients with watch-and-wait had a significantly better overall score, and significant betters scores in the specific sectors of liquid and gas continence and the need for a continence pad.

The study by van der Sande et al.[25] examined anorectal function in rectal cancer patients following a watch-and-wait policy after chemoradiotherapy and undertook to investigate the dose–volume effects of radiotherapy on anorectal function at two years. Thirty-three patients with primary rectal cancer who were treated with chemoradiotherapy and a watch-and-wait policy with minimum follow-up of two years were included. They assessed anorectal function using anorectal manometry and patient-reported outcomes (Vaizey and LARS score). Median dose of radiation to the rectum and anal sphincter complex was 50.5 Gy and 44.7 Gy, respectively. After a median follow-up of 38 (range 23–116) months, 33.3% of the patients reported major LARS. The mean LARS score was 23.4 ± 11.3 and the mean Vaizey score was 4.3 ± 4.1. The most frequent complaints were clustering of defaecation and faecal urgency. There was also a non-significant trend towards a higher Vaizey and LARS score after a higher anal sphincter complex dose.

What you choose to measure, and in whom and how, will determine your results, and as such, interpretation of the results of the presently available data needs to be carefully considered. The studies so far are heterogeneous and generally report only short–term follow-up. They have had different QoL assessments at different times, and of patients who had a variety of different cancer stages and different treatment regimes. The QoL assessments have focused heavily on anorectal function. Despite this, these studies show the following generalizable points:

1. Patients who have an excellent response to CRT and continue the OP pathway have better bowel, urological and sexual function and resultant better QoL across several domains compared with those who have TME (with or without CRT).
2. Patients with unsuccessful OP (i.e. those who had CRT for early stage rectal cancer then proceeded to TME) can be expected to have worse function and QoL than those who had TME alone.
3. Patients who have successful OP have some impairment of rectal (and likely urological and sexual) function, and some develop LARS, though at a lesser rate than those who have a TME (with or without CRT).

References

1. Cella DF, Tulsky DS. Measuring quality of life today: methodological aspects: Oncology (Williston Park, N.Y.). 1990;4(5):29–38; discussion 69).
2. Sajid M, Tonsi A, Baig M. Health-related quality of life measurement. *Int J Health Care Qual Assur*. 2008;21(4):365–73.
3. Ghosh RK, Ghosh SM, Ganguly G. Health-related quality of life and its growing importance in clinical practice. *N Z Med J*. 2010;123(1313):99–101.
4. Carr AJ, Higginson IJ. Are quality of life measures patient centred?. *BMJ*. 2001;322(7298):1357–60.
5. Marventano S, Forjaz M, Grosso G, et al. Health related quality of life in colorectal cancer patients: state of the art. *BMC Surg*. 2013;13(2):1–7
6. Herdman M, Gudex C, Lloyd A, et al. Development and preliminary testing of the new five-level version of EQ-5D (EQ-5D-5L). *Qual Life Res*. 2011;20(10):1727–36.
7. Ware J, Kosinski M, Keller S. A 12-item short-form health survey: construction of scales and preliminary tests of reliability and validity. *Med Care*. 1996;34(3):220–33.
8. Whistance RN, Conroy T, Chie W, et al. Clinical and psychometric validation of the EORTC QLQ-CR29 questionnaire module to assess health-related quality of life in patients with colorectal cancer. *Eur J Cancer*. 2009;45(17):3017–26.
9. Ward WL1, Hahn EA, Mo F, Hernandez L, Tulsky DS, Cella D. Reliability and validity of the Functional Assessment of Cancer Therapy-Colorectal (FACT-C) quality of life instrument. *Qual Life Res*. 1999;8(3):181–95.
10. Ring L, Höfer S, Heuston F, Harris D, O'Boyle CA. Response shift masks the treatment impact on patient reported outcomes (PROs): the example of individual quality of life in edentulous patients. *Health Qual Life Outcomes*. 2005 7(3):55.
11. Kind P, Lafata JE, Matuszewski K, Raisch D. The use of QALYs in clinical and patient decision-making: issues and prospects. *Value Health*. 2009; 12 Suppl 1:S27–30.
12. Sprangers MAG, Schwartz CE. Integrating response shift into health-related quality of life research: a theoretical model. *Soc Sci Med*. 1999;48(11):1507–15.
13. Kollmotgen CF, Meagher AP, Wolff BG, Pemberton JH, Martenson JA, Illstrup DM, the long term effects of adjuvant postoperative chemoradiation for rectal cancer on bowel function. *Ann Surg*. 1994;220(5):676–82
14. Croese AD, Lonie JM, Trollope AF, Vangaveti VN, Ho YH. A meta-analysis of the prevalence of low anterior resection syndrome and systematic review of risk factors. *Int J Surg*. 2018;56:234–41.

15. Ho YH, Seow-Choen F, Tan M. Colonic J-pouch function at six months versus straight coloanal anastomosis at two years: randomized controlled trial. *World J Surg.* 2001;25:876–81.
16. Lazorthes F, Chiotasso P, Gamagami RA, Istvan G, Chevreau P. Late clinical outcome in a randomized prospective comparison of colonic J pouch and straight coloanal anastomosis. *Br J Surg.* 1997;84:1449–51.
17. Bregendahl S, Emmertsen KJ, Lous J, Laurberg S. Bowel dysfunction after low anterior resection with and without neoadjuvant therapy for rectal cancer: a population-based cross-sectional study. *Colorectal Dis.* 2013;15:1130–9.
18. Chen TY, Wiltink LM, Nout RA, Meershoek-Klein Kranenbarg E, Laurberg S, Marijnen CA, van de Velde CJ. Bowel function 14 years after preoperative short-course radiotherapy and total mesorectal excision for rectal cancer: report of a multicenter randomized trial. *Clin Colorectal Cancer.* 2015;14:106–14.
19. Kupsch J, Jackisch T, Matzel KE, et al. Outcome of bowel function following anterior resection for rectal cancer-an analysis using the low anterior resection syndrome (LARS) score. *Int J Colorectal Dis.* 2018;33:787–98.
20. Kupsch J, Kuhn M, Matzel KE, et al. To what extent is the low anterior resection syndrome (LARS) associated with quality of life as measured using the EORTC C30 and CR38 quality of life questionnaires? *Int J Colorectal Dis.* 2019;34:747–62.
21. Habr-Gama A, Lynn PB, Jorge JM, São Julião GP, Proscurshim I, Gama-Rodrigues J, Fernandez LM, Perez RO. Impact of organ-preserving strategies on anorectal function in patients with distal rectal cancer following neoadjuvant chemoradiation. *Dis Colon Rectum.* 2016;59(4):264–9.
22. Hupkens BJP, Martens MH, Stoot JH, et al. Quality of life in rectal cancer patients after chemoradiation: watch-and-wait policy versus standard resection—a matched-controlled study. *Dis Colon Rectum.* 2017;60(10):1032–40.
23. Lynn PB, Renfro LA, Carrero XW, Shi Q, Strombom PL, Chow O, Garcia-Aguilar J. Anorectal function and quality of life in patients with early stage rectal cancer treated with chemoradiation and local excision. *Dis Colon Rectum.* 2017;60(5):459–68.
24. Martens MH, Maas M, Heijnen LA, et al. Long-term outcome of an organ preservation program after neoadjuvant treatment for rectal cancer. *J Natl Cancer Inst.* 2016;108(12):djw171.
25. van der Sande ME, Hupkens BJP, Berbée M, et al. Impact of radiotherapy on anorectal function in patients with rectal cancer following a watch and wait programme. *Radiother Oncol.* 2019;132:79–84.

14

Tumouroids and patient-specific responses in rectal cancer

Kasmira C. Wilson, Lloyd Pereira, Robert G. Ramsay, and Alexander G. Heriot

Background

There has been increasing enthusiasm in organ preservation for rectal cancer patients who achieve a complete clinical response (cCR) to neo-adjuvant therapy. This approach has been championed by Habr-Gama with a 2004 publication of rectal cancer patients treated with chemoradiotherapy (CRT) followed by a 'watch and wait approach'.[1] Due to the unpredictability of individual responses to CRT organ preservation needs to be tailored to clinical response. Neo-adjuvant chemoradiotherapy (NACRT) for locally advanced rectal cancer followed by total mesorectal excision has traditionally been considered the standard of care, with recommendation for adjuvant chemotherapy directed by TNM staging.[2,3] A complete pathological response is achieved in around 20% of patients, the remaining patients either achieve a partial or no response to therapy.[4] Patients with a genuine pathological complete response have more favourable outcomes.[4]

More recently there has been a shift toward the delivery of total neoadjuvant therapy (TNT) for patients with locally advanced rectal cancers.[5] This has demonstrated pCR rates of around 30%,[6,7] and facilitated higher rates of organ preservation.

Despite the therapy approach there remains no current method to delineate which patients are likely to respond to neo-adjuvant therapy, thus re-staging needs to be completed before a favourable response is known. Given this the opportunity to offer organ preservation to patients with rectal cancer is unpredictable and relies on what has been described as an 'incidental' complete response.[8] Fundamentally this makes it impractical to tailor treatment options to individual patients and limits the delivery of patient-specific therapies in rectal cancer. Response to NACRT is assessed by clinical examination, with no identification of residual tumour considered a complete clinical response (cCR). However, this can be difficult to diagnose. There is also no standard consensus on what factors are required for the diagnosis of a cCR.[9] Ideally, a cCR would be used as a surrogate for a pCR in therapy, however; the identification of a cCR on re-staging does not always correlate with a histopathological assessment of a pCR on resected specimens.[10]

Despite the limitations in correlating a cCR with a pCR, the selection of patients whom may benefit from a 'watch and wait' approach has proven feasible and safe.[11] A meta-analysis has demonstrated the three year cumulative risk of local regrowth is 21.6 %, with most of these cases amenable to salvage surgery, with three year overall survival of 93.5%.[12] Patients whom are candidates for 'watch and wait' regimes would be expected to have excellent outcomes with surgery, it is therefore important to note that there is worse survival and a higher incidence of distant progression in these patients who have a local regrowth when compared to those without local regrowth.[13] This is likely a reflection of disease biology, rather than a consequence of organ preservation. This again highlights the imperative requirement to develop innovative techniques to assist with patient selection and enable precision direction of treatment.[14]

Tumour models

'Benchtop to bedside research' is championed as one of the bolsters necessary to achieve precision oncology. Several cancer models have previously been pioneered and utilized and these have proven indispensable in obtaining detailed knowledge around tumour development, stasis, and evolution. However, these models have been unable to completely recapitulate *in-vivo* tumour pathophysiology.

Cell lines have been a model long utilized in cancer research, with tumour cells originally established as a cell line as early as 1951.[15] Cell lines have gone on to become common models used to research cancer due to their unlimited supply, favourable ethical profile, reproducibility, manipulability, and drug-screening capabilities. Cell lines do not retain the native architecture of the original tumour and lack three-dimensional cell interactions. The tumour microenvironment and structural components, which are known to influence cellular biology, are also lacking. As cell lines are passaged on artificial substrates, genetic drift occurs, leading to phenotypic and genotypic variations compared to the native tumour.[16] With this in mind, cell lines have been demonstrated to be of limited use in studying various physiological processes.[17] It is also now recognized that cells cultured in two-dimensional conditions may have altered signalling pathways when compared to *in-vivo* conditions.[18] Understandably then cell lines have not been high-yielding in predicting how the *in-vivo* tumour will respond to therapy.

Animal models have proven to be another common cancer therapy testing platform. Due to evolutionary conservation, mice have a significant genetic overlap with humans.[19] Mouse platforms have been extensively utilized as cancer models, and can be selectively manipulated genetically or employed to create a patient-derived xenograft platform to replicate *in-vivo* conditions.[20] Again, despite the enthusiasm to use these models, results have not correlated with responses.[21]

Ideal models for studying tumour demand pathophysiological representation of the tumour, including vascularization and immune components, the ability to facilitate high-throughput screening, manipulability, the option for biobanking, genome editing, and disease modelling.[22] In order to achieve these desired features, we need to look beyond traditional models and assess unfolding advances in tissue culture techniques that may aid the development of this 'holy grail' model.

Organoids

The need to move beyond monolayer cell culture techniques to include elements of the extracellular matrix and reconstitute the tumour microenvironment has been well recognized. Three-dimensional culture techniques have been pioneered since 1989 by Barcellos-Hoff.[23] More recently, other studies have demonstrated the ability of stem cells derived from the adult intestine to self-organize *in* vitro.[24] This research has since been expanded to establish intestinal organoids that maintain the structure of their tissue of origin, and all four intestinal cell types of the small intestinal crypt.[25]

Organoids are essentially mini organs that are cultured *in vitro*. They are derived from stem cells and are comprised of numerous cell types that are self-organizing and resemble many components of the organ in terms of physiology and cellular interactions.[26] It was promptly realized that this technology provided a platform to study not only the physiology of normal tissue, but also pathological disease processes, including tumour formation and physiology.[22] Organoids can be derived from small tissue biopsies of normal tissue, *in situ* tumours (tumouroids) or resectional specimens. Because organoids are derived from stem cells, they are able to recapitulate the heterogenicity of both parental and tumour cells.[27] Once established organoids are self-renewing allowing the generation of adequate material for research purposes, this has propelled the publication of expansive literature across multiple tumour streams.[22]

The technique of deriving organoids from intestinal tissue is well established and has been optimized to derive organoids from colonic tissue and tumouroids from colorectal cancers. Intestinal stem cells reside within intestinal crypts and renew the intestinal epithelium. As intestinal stem cells proliferate in the crypts, they respond to growth factors secreted by surrounding cell populations. As these cells migrate upward from the crypt base, they differentiate into the cell populations that comprise the intestinal epithelium. LGR5 has been demonstrated as a marker of the intestinal stem-cell population.[28] These LGR5 positive cells expand and differentiate into the cells found in the intestinal epithelium, validating this population of cells as a multipotent adult intestinal stem cell.[29] Organoids generated from the LGR5-positive cell population have been further shown to recapitulate the structure of the intestinal epithelium and maintain the diverse cell populations present.[28]

Identification of the specific markers that define intestinal stem-cell populations has allowed a deepened understanding of the mechanisms that underpin stem-cell-driven homeostasis of the intestine. Broadening this research has also provided added insights into how this impacts the formation of intestinal cancers.[29] When considering rectal cancer, it is important to highlight that colonic stem cells have also been identified. This was done by identifying a population of cells positive for EPHB2 expression.[30] These EPHB2 positive cells have also been propagated using three-dimensional culture techniques and found to differentiate into the three predominant cell populations found in the colonic epithelium, thus providing an *in-vitro* model of the human colon.[30]

The methods underpinning the generation of tumouroids derived from rectal tumours are relatively straightforward. Tumour tissue is obtained either from biopsies of the tumour *in situ* or from the resected specimen. Tumour tissue is then dissected into small pieces and digested to form a single-cell suspension. The digested cellular suspension contains colonic stem cells, which are then implanted into a soluble matrix such as Matrigel®. Matrigel® is derived from mouse sarcoma cells and is designed to reconstitute the basement membrane and provide an extracellular matrix for the establishment of these stem-cell-derived tumouroids.[31] Once stem cells are embedded into this three-dimensional matrix, media containing appropriate growth factors is added, and cells are incubated in conditions that mimic those observed *in vivo.* Stem cells derived from the rectal tumour grow and expand into rectal tumouroid models (Fig. 14.1).

The selection of growth factors incorporated into the media is dependent on the type of organoid or tumouroid being cultured. In the setting of rectal cancer tumouroids, these factors are designed to support and promote tumourigenesis. Established cultures can then be maintained under conditions that replicate aspects of the tumour microenvironment with easy control of factors such as temperature and hypoxia. Stem cells in this culture proliferate and self-organize to then form the

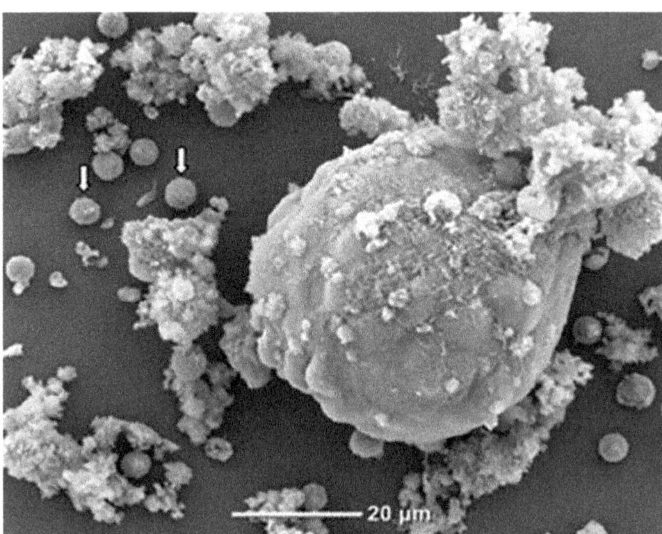

Fig. 14.1 Electron scanning microscopy image of a rectal tumouroid co-cultured with patient-matched tumour-infiltrating lymphocytes (arrows).

differentiated cell populations observed in the parental tumour. Genetic expression analysis of tumouroids cultivated under these conditions has demonstrated them to be a robust long-term preclinical culture model that accurately replicates the parental tumour phenotypically, genotypically, and morphologically.[30]

Three-dimensional tumouroid models have been instrumental in a boom of projects researching drug development, immunology, toxicology, and oncology.[32] Using the culturing techniques outlined earlier, there is now the capacity to create a three-dimensional, multicellular model that incorporates cell-to-cell interactions and maintains functional features, as well as models the structure of the extracellular matrix. To build upon this development and more accurately replicate *in-vivo* conditions, this culture technique can be amplified to allow the addition of stromal components or cells derived from other sources, allowing multiple facets of tumourigenesis and tumour immunology to be explored. The self-regenerating component of this model mimics the advantages highlighted with cell lines, and allows the expansion of individual lines of tumouroids derived from multiple sources including from the gastro-intestinal tract, to create tumouroid banks.[33,34]

Utilization of tumouroid models

Tumouroid models have provided a foundation for a vast array of research methods (Fig. 14.2). Drug and compound testing has long been limited by the lack of concordance between results obtained from cell lines and animal models. Toxicity profiles cannot be extrapolated reliably from these models. It is therefore important to have an improved human-based system to facilitate rapid drug testing, which can not only identify drugs that may be of therapeutic value, but also assess the toxicity of these drugs. Organoids may indeed be the tipping point in allowing full realization of this. Organoids have also been demonstrated to express drug transporters and maintain efflux transport activity as well as the ability to induce drug-metabolizing enzymes,[35] leading to an interest in their ability to be used as models to assess the pharmacokinetics of drugs. The ability to concurrently grow organoids from normal tissue in addition to those derived from tumour tissue provides a platform for the comparison of toxicity between normal and tumour cells. This information could direct dosing models to target tumour cells but maintain the viability of cells in disease-free sites.

Mouse-derived tumouroids were identified to be more accurate predictors of *in-vivo* response to chemotherapeutic therapy (5FU) when compared to colorectal cell lines.[36] Drug testing using human tumouroid models is currently underway, with colorectal cancer tumouroids already validated in an automated high-throughput platform for drug testing.[37] The ability to expand large numbers of tumouroids from patient tissue allows tumouroids to be tested against a vast number of different compounds at different concentrations in a single run. However, it is not simply enough to confirm that these models can be utilized for drug testing, it is also necessary to prove that this technique models the *in-vivo* patient response to therapy, allowing them to

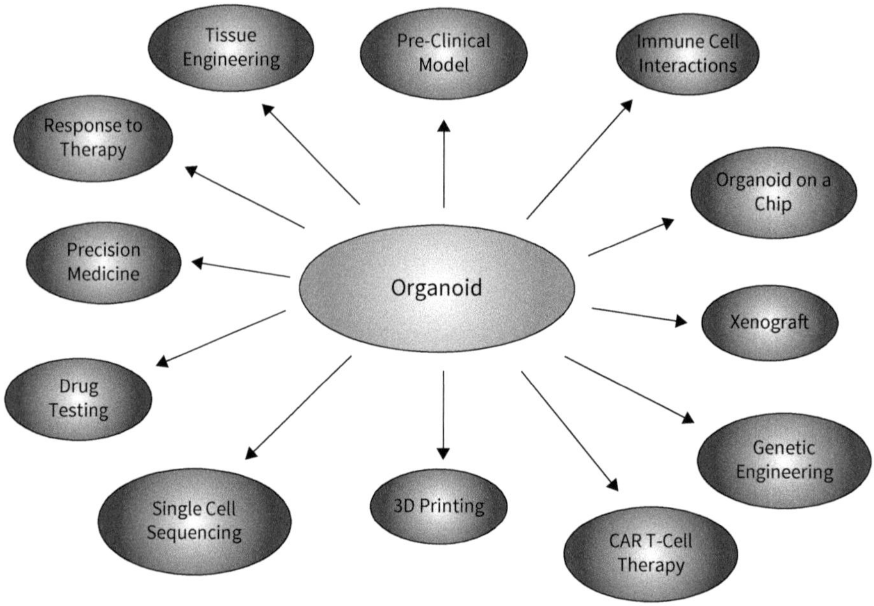

Fig. 14.2 Current research applications that utilize organoids include the culture of patient-derived organoids or tumouroids for use as a preclinical model,[32] which provides a platform for rapid drug testing and to explore the immune landscape of tumours,[56,65] as well as to predict patient response to therapy.[62] Further utilization has occurred in xenograft models,[20] and organoid on a chip technology[70] as well as in association with chimeric antigen receptor-engineered lymphocytes.[59] Organoid and tumouroid technology has provided platforms that facilitate genetic engineering,[55] tissue engineering and 3D bioprinting techniques.[48,71] These models have also enabled single-cell sequencing,[27] and assisted in the establishment of platforms to deliver precision medicine.[43]

be validated as a predictive model. Accurate prediction of response to therapy has been confirmed across multiple tumour types with gastric tumouroids.[38] These results demonstrate the potential of using tumouroids to tailor therapy for individual patients including the ability to test the effects of novel drugs and compounds or assess the utility of repurposing existing therapies. High-throughput drug testing of colorectal tumouroids has proven feasible and further work in this area may realize this as a validated method for treatment selection.[39,40] As tumouroids replicate the response of native tissue, they also provide the opportunity to study mechanisms that confer resistance to therapy, allowing a deeper exploration of why individuals express such varied treatment responses.[41]

Tumouroids have been used in parallel to patient therapy to assess how accurately the observed *in-vitro* responses to therapy mimic the *in-vivo* patient responses to therapy.[42] Gastrointestinal tumouroid models have been used to demonstrate that tumouroids have the ability to recapitulate the response observed in the parental tumour, validating this as a preclinical model for drug testing.[43] To recreate a more accurate representation of the *in-vivo* conditions, additional cells can be added into culture conditions.[44] The immune response to colorectal cancer has been shown to be an important predictor of patient response to drug therapy and immune infiltrates have been validated as a prognostic tool for patients with colorectal cancer.[45] Patient-derived tumouroids have been established with immune cell populations maintained in culture, immune profiling of these cultured cells demonstrated that there was preservation of immune cell subsets between the tumouroid culture and the native tumour tissue, providing an avenue to more extensively explore aspects of the tumour microenvironment.[46]

Co-culture techniques are not limited to cells of the immune system, with assays pioneering the addition of neuronal cells and fibroblasts to organoid cultures.[47] Tissue engineering has resulted in the generation of organoids with a functional enteric nervous system.[48] Additionally, a fusion of models has been created with human-derived organoids implanted into mice and supported by mouse vasculature.[49] These models seek to accurately represent *in-vivo* conditions, capturing all aspects of tumourigenesis. Tumouroids have also been utilized to explore the metastatic cascade by characterizing the signalling pathway involved in the early stages of metastasis. This was achieved by engineering a colorectal cancer model to create a manipulatable stroma compartment, allowing the incorporation of vascularized stroma in the culture and the analysis of angiogenic factors.[50] Further advances in this field include the ongoing development of tissue culture techniques, where the evolution of different substrates is used to model the extracellular matrix. While Matrigel® has proven invaluable in the design of three-dimensional culture techniques, it is relatively fixed in structure and does not accurately model the biomechanical forces that occur *in vivo*. Hybrid and designer matrices have thus been developed to address these issues.[51] Tissue engineering of matrices has also allowed additional cells to be incorporated that reconstitute a more physiological representation of the extracellular matrix.[52,53]

Genomic assessment of tumour tissue has long held hope to be able to predict response to therapy in rectal cancer, but this expectation has not yet been realized despite significant advances in the field. Organoids and tumouroids are amenable to genetic engineering as well as single-cell sequencing techniques. CRISPR-Cas9 genetic engineering allows the modification of selected genes with predesigned mutations. CRISPR editing of tumouroids has been instrumental in evolving the understanding of underlying molecular mechanisms that contribute to the formation of colorectal tumours.[54] This technology has recently been used on xenograft mouse model-derived tumouroids to validate colorectal cancer driver genes.[55]

In addition to using genetics to explore the oncogenic process, genetic interrogation of hepatocytes has allowed the identification of bipotent liver progenitors that can be utilized to generate organoids. These organoids can subsequently be expanded *in vitro* and transplanted into mouse models with the aim of reversing pathological processes.[56] Genetic engineering of lymphocytes is a well-described form of immunotherapy now invaluable for the treatment of patients with leukaemia.[57] These chimeric antigen receptor-engineered lymphocytes (CAR-T cells) have been used *in vitro* against tumouroid models of disease to assess the value of this therapy in targeting colorectal tumours.[58,59] Advances in next-generating sequencing platforms and single-cell genomics has provided an additional platform to assess colorectal tumouroid responses to oxaliplatin on a single-cell scale.[27] Adding a further layer of interrogation of the utility of tumouroids as a model for drug testing and response. Single-cell sequencing has also been utilized to understand the contribution of the microenvironment to tumouroid culture models.[60]

The role of tumouroids in rectal cancer

Organoids and tumouroids have exciting implications for oncology as highlighted by their recent use in multidrug testing.[43] Tumouroids derived from a patient with treatment-refractory metastatic colorectal cancer have been used to direct second-line chemotherapy.[61] The specific application of tumouroids to rectal cancer is limited. Rectal cancer tumouroids can be established from tissue biopsies in as little as two weeks (Fig. 14.3). A novel culture approach combining patient-derived

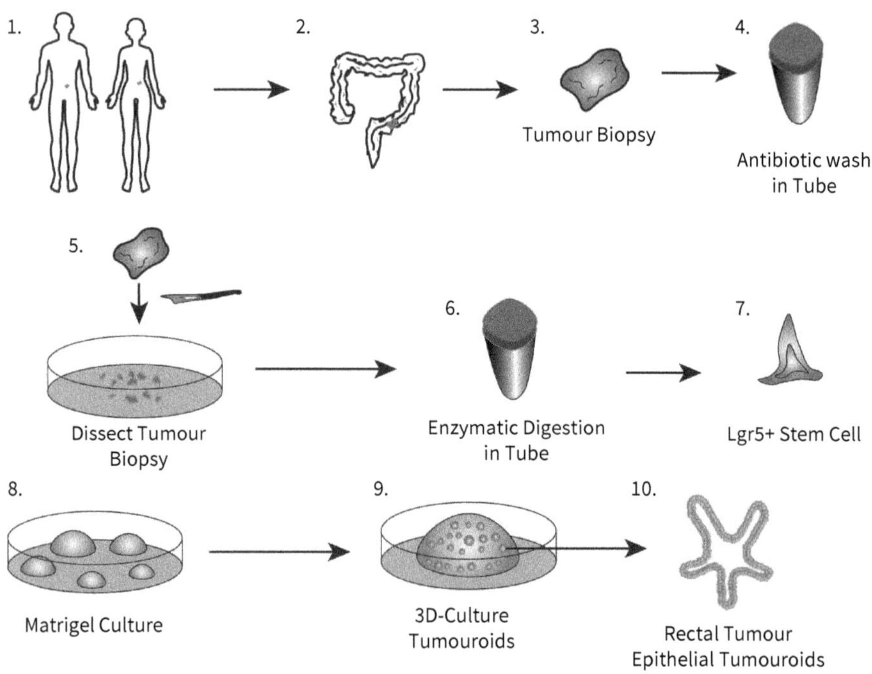

Fig. 14.3 Generation of patient-derived rectal cancer tumouroids from an endoscopic biopsy of rectal tumour tissue. Tumour biopsies are washed in antibiotic media prior to dissection into small tumour pieces. This dissected tissue is digested into a single-cell suspension and then implanted into a Matrigel® dome. Culture with media containing appropriate growth factors allows the establishment of rectal cancer tumouroids.

tumour-infiltrating lymphocytes (TILs) in co-culture with patient-derived rectal tumouroids has been established.[62] This platform has been used to move beyond drug testing, instead focusing on the ability to utilize tumouroids as a tool to explore the role of anti-tumour immunity in relation to NACRT. This assay has demonstrated the ability to predict responses to NACRT in a clinically relevant timeframe.[62] Patients with T3 to T4 and/or N1 to N2 locally advanced rectal cancers were recruited to the study. Patients were required to undergo long-course NACRT, followed by surgery, with 17 patients completing the intended treatment, and having tumouroids and TILs generated from pretreatment biopsies. Patients with a complete pathological response to neo-adjuvant therapy had enhanced cytotoxicity of their tumouroids by $CD8^+$ T cells when compared to patients who had no response to therapy. Thus, TIL function has been utilized as a biomarker for response to NACRT.[62] While this is a small study, the fact that it has demonstrated the ability to predict response to NACRT has substantive potential implications. A validated assay that accurately predicts response has significant opportunities in this field and could be used as a tool to select patients who would be candidates for 'watch and wait' surveillance and organ preservation.

Immunotherapy has been championed as the 'fourth pillar' in oncology alongside surgery, radiotherapy, and chemotherapy. The role of immunotherapy to target rectal tumours has not been well defined outside of patients presenting with microsatellite (MSI) unstable tumours.[63,64] It is undeniable that immunotherapy in the form of checkpoint inhibition has generated impressive results in mismatch repair-deficient rectal cancer.[64] Notably, MSI high tumours are more frequently associated with right-sided colon cancers and are relatively uncommon in rectal tumours.[65] Therefore, further exploration of the role of anti-tumoural immunity in targeting rectal cancer is warranted. Tumouroids maintain a mutational load that overlaps significantly with the tumour of origin,[43] identifying them as a valuable tool in the exploration of tumour immunity. This provides the opportunity for further applications of this platform to assess the role of immunotherapy in the treatment of rectal cancer, as tumouroid response to immune checkpoint therapy has been correlated to tumour response in other tumour streams.[66]

Future directions of tumouroid models in rectal cancer

The potential for tumouroids to be used for rapid drug-screening and prediction of response to NACRT has been outlined. Currently patient-derived tumouroids are being collated into biobanks to provide resources for future avenues of study including genomics.[34] It is now accepted that tumouroids reflect the characteristics of the native tumour and provide an avenue for in-depth molecular analysis.[67] Characterization of the mutational pathways leading to tumourigenesis as well as resistance to standard therapies will facilitate the identification of potential new drug targets, and biomarkers.

The ability to model carcinogenesis *in vitro* has also provided the opportunity to study mutations leading to metastasis in colon cancer, specifically in relation to niche factor dependency.[68] This technology has the potential to be translated to rectal tumouroids to further understand mechanisms underlying metastasis.

Next generation organoid technology is poised to utilize organoid-on-a-chip technology to evaluate the interplay between the *in situ* tumour and environmental substrates and cells. Further aspects of signalling relating to the extracellular environment, including the role of mechanical forces in signalling, can thus be explored in the setting of rectal cancer.[69] Tissue culture of organoids incorporating CRISPR gene editing techniques, as well as engineered CAR-T cells specific to rectal tumours have the potential to further explore novel targeted therapies.

References

1. Habr-Gama A, Perez RO, Nadalin W, et al. Operative versus nonoperative treatment for stage 0 distal rectal cancer following chemoradiation therapy: long-term results. *Ann Surg.* 2004;240(4):711–17; discussion 717–18.
2. Bregni G, Akin Telli T, Camera S, et al. Adjuvant chemotherapy for rectal cancer: Current evidence and recommendations for clinical practice. *Cancer Treat Rev.* 2020;83:101948.
3. Chen M, Chen LZ, Xu L, Zhang JS, Song X. Neoadjuvant chemoradiation for locally advanced rectal cancer: a systematic review of the literature with network meta-analysis. *Cancer Manag Res.* 2019;11:741–58.
4. Maas M, Nelemans PJ, Valentini V, et al. Long-term outcome in patients with a pathological complete response after chemoradiation for rectal cancer: a pooled analysis of individual patient data. *Lancet Oncol.* 2010;11(9):835–44.
5. Garcia-Aguilar J, Patil S, Gollub MJ, et al. Organ Preservation in patients with rectal adenocarcinoma treated with total neoadjuvant therapy. *J Clin Oncol.* 2022;40(23):2546–56.
6. Bahadoer RR, Dijkstra EA, van Etten B, et al. Short-course radiotherapy followed by chemotherapy before total mesorectal excision (TME) versus preoperative chemoradiotherapy, TME, and optional adjuvant chemotherapy in locally advanced rectal cancer (RAPIDO): a randomised, open-label, phase 3 trial. *Lancet Oncol.* 2021;22(1):29–42.
7. Conroy T, Bosset JF, Etienne PL, et al. Neoadjuvant chemotherapy with FOLFIRINOX and preoperative chemoradiotherapy for patients with locally advanced rectal cancer (UNICANCER-PRODIGE 23): a multicentre, randomised, open-label, phase 3 trial. *Lancet Oncol.* 2021;22(5):702–15.
8. Gani C, Kirschniak A, Zips D. Watchful Waiting after Radiochemotherapy in Rectal Cancer: When Is It Feasible? *Visc Med.* 2019;35(2):119–23.
9. Couch DG, Hemingway DM. Complete radiotherapy response in rectal cancer: A review of the evidence. *World J Gastroenterol.* 2016;22(2):467–70.
10. Creavin B, Ryan E, Martin ST, et al. Organ preservation with local excision or active surveillance following chemoradiotherapy for rectal cancer. *Br J Cancer.* 2017;116(2):169–74.
11. Maas M, Beets-Tan RG, Lambregts DM, et al. Wait-and-see policy for clinical complete responders after chemoradiation for rectal cancer. *J Clin Oncol.* 2011;29(35):4633–40.
12. Dattani M, Heald RJ, Goussous G, et al. Oncological and survival outcomes in watch and wait patients with a clinical complete response after neoadjuvant chemoradiotherapy for rectal cancer: a systematic review and pooled analysis. *Ann Surg.* 2018;268(6):955–67.

13. Smith JJ, Strombom P, Chow OS, et al. Assessment of a watch-and-wait strategy for rectal cancer in patients with a complete response after neoadjuvant therapy. *JAMA Oncol.* 2019;5:e185896.
14. Ryan JE, Warrier SK, Lynch AC, Heriot AG. Assessing pathological complete response to neoadjuvant chemoradiotherapy in locally advanced rectal cancer: a systematic review. *Colorectal Dis.* 2015;17(10):849–61.
15. Scherer WF, Syverton JT, Gey GO. Studies on the propagation in vitro of poliomyelitis viruses. IV. Viral multiplication in a stable strain of human malignant epithelial cells (strain HeLa) derived from an epidermoid carcinoma of the cervix. *J Exp Med.* 1953;97(5):695–710.
16. Nestor CE, Ottaviano R, Reinhardt D, et al. Rapid reprogramming of epigenetic and transcriptional profiles in mammalian culture systems. *Genome Biol.* 2015;16:11.
17. Jenkinson SE, Chung GW, van Loon E, Bakar NS, Dalzell AM, Brown CD. The limitations of renal epithelial cell line HK-2 as a model of drug transporter expression and function in the proximal tubule. *Pflugers Arch.* 2012;464(6):601–11.
18. Wang F, Weaver VM, Petersen OW, et al. Reciprocal interactions between beta1-integrin and epidermal growth factor receptor in three-dimensional basement membrane breast cultures: a different perspective in epithelial biology. *Proc Natl Acad Sci U S A.* 1998;95(25):14821–6.
19. Mural RJ, Adams MD, Myers EW, et al. A comparison of whole-genome shotgun-derived mouse chromosome 16 and the human genome. *Science.* 2002;296(5573):1661–71.
20. Bleijs M, van de Wetering M, Clevers H, Drost J. Xenograft and organoid model systems in cancer research. *EMBO J.* 2019;*38*(15):e101654.
21. Johnson JI, Decker S, Zaharevitz D, et al. Relationships between drug activity in NCI preclinical in vitro and in vivo models and early clinical trials. *Br J Cancer.* 2001;84(10):1424–31.
22. Li M, Izpisua Belmonte JC. Organoids - Preclinical Models of Human Disease. *N Engl J Med.* 2019;380(6):569–79.
23. Barcellos-Hoff MH, Aggeler J, Ram TG, Bissell MJ. Functional differentiation and alveolar morphogenesis of primary mammary cultures on reconstituted basement membrane. *Development.* 1989;105(2):223–35.
24. Sato T, van Es JH, Snippert HJ, et al. Paneth cells constitute the niche for Lgr5 stem cells in intestinal crypts. *Nature.* 2011;469(7330):415–18.
25. Drost J, Clevers H. Organoids in cancer research. *Nat Rev Cancer.* 2018;18(7):407–18.
26. Lancaster MA, Knoblich JA. Organogenesis in a dish: modeling development and disease using organoid technologies. *Science.* 2014;345(6194):1247125.
27. Chen KY, Srinivasan T, Lin C, et al. Single-Cell Transcriptomics Reveals Heterogeneity and Drug Response of Human Colorectal Cancer Organoids. *Conf Proc IEEE Eng Med Biol Soc.* 2018;2018:2378–81.
28. Sato T, Vries RG, Snippert HJ, et al. Single Lgr5 stem cells build crypt-villus structures in vitro without a mesenchymal niche. *Nature.* 2009;459(7244):262–65.
29. Barker N. Adult intestinal stem cells: critical drivers of epithelial homeostasis and regeneration. *Nat Rev Mol Cell Biol.* 2014;15(1):19–33.
30. Jung P, Sato T, Merlos-Suarez A, et al. Isolation and in vitro expansion of human colonic stem cells. *Nat Med.* 2011;17(10):1225–7.
31. Kleinman HK, Martin GR. Matrigel: basement membrane matrix with biological activity. *Semin Cancer Biol.* 2005;15(5):378–86.
32. Singh A, Nikkhah M, Annabi N. Biomaterials, Cells, and Patho-physiology: Building Better Organoids and On-Chip Technologies. *Biomaterials.* 2019;198:1–2.

33. Saito Y. Establishment of an organoid bank of biliary tract and pancreatic cancers and its application for personalized therapy and future treatment. *J Gastroenterol Hepatol.* 2019;*34*:1906–10.
34. van de Wetering M, Francies HE, Francis JM, et al. Prospective derivation of a living organoid biobank of colorectal cancer patients. *Cell.* 7 2015;161(4):933–45.
35. Onozato D, Yamashita M, Nakanishi A, et al. Generation of intestinal organoids suitable for pharmacokinetic studies from human induced pluripotent stem cells. *Drug Metab Dispos.* 2018;46(11):1572–80.
36. Grabinger T, Luks L, Kostadinova F, et al. Ex vivo culture of intestinal crypt organoids as a model system for assessing cell death induction in intestinal epithelial cells and enteropathy. *Cell Death Dis.* 2014;5:e1228.
37. Boehnke K, Iversen PW, Schumacher D, et al. Assay Establishment and Validation of a High-Throughput Screening Platform for Three-Dimensional Patient-Derived Colon Cancer Organoid Cultures. *J Biomol Screen.* 2016;21(9):931–41.
38. Steele NG, Chakrabarti J, Wang J, et al. An Organoid-Based Preclinical Model of Human Gastric Cancer. *Cell Mol Gastroenterol Hepatol.* 2019;7(1):161–84.
39. He X, Jiang Y, Zhang L, et al. Patient-derived organoids as a platform for drug screening in metastatic colorectal cancer. *Front Bioeng Biotechnol.* 2023;11:1190637.
40. Tan T, Mouradov D, Gibbs P, Sieber OM. Protocol for generation of and high-throughput drug testing with patient-derived colorectal cancer organoids. *STAR Protoc.* 2024;5(2):103090.
41. Plodinec M, Schoenenberger CA. Spatial organization acts on cell signaling: how physical force contributes to the development of cancer. *Breast Cancer Res.* 2010;12(4):308.
42. Flood M, Narasimhan V, Wilson K, et al. Organoids as a Robust Preclinical Model for Precision Medicine in Colorectal Cancer: A Systematic Review. *Ann Surg Oncol.* 2021;29(1):47–59.
43. Vlachogiannis G, Hedayat S, Vatsiou A, et al. Patient-derived organoids model treatment response of metastatic gastrointestinal cancers. *Science.* 2018;359(6378):920–6.
44. Nozaki K, Mochizuki W, Matsumoto Y, et al. Co-culture with intestinal epithelial organoids allows efficient expansion and motility analysis of intraepithelial lymphocytes. *J Gastroenterol.* 2016;51(3):206–13.
45. Pages F, Mlecnik B, Marliot F, et al. International validation of the consensus Immunoscore for the classification of colon cancer: a prognostic and accuracy study. *Lancet.* 2018;391(10135):2128–39.
46. Neal JT, Li X, Zhu J, et al. Organoid Modeling of the Tumor Immune Microenvironment. *Cell.* 2018;175(7):1972–88 e1916.
47. Pastula A, Middelhoff M, Brandtner A, et al. Three-Dimensional Gastrointestinal Organoid Culture in Combination with Nerves or Fibroblasts: A Method to Characterize the Gastrointestinal Stem Cell Niche. *Stem Cells Int.* 2016;2016:3710836.
48. Workman MJ, Mahe MM, Trisno S, et al. Engineered human pluripotent-stem-cell-derived intestinal tissues with a functional enteric nervous system. *Nat Med.* 2017;23(1):49–59.
49. Watson CL, Mahe MM, Munera J, et al. An in vivo model of human small intestine using pluripotent stem cells. *Nat Med.* 2014;20(11):1310–14.
50. Pape J, Magdeldin T, Ali M, et al. Cancer invasion regulates vascular complexity in a three-dimensional biomimetic model. *Eur J Cancer.* 2019;119:179–93.
51. Gjorevski N, Sachs N, Manfrin A, et al. Designer matrices for intestinal stem cell and organoid culture. *Nature.* 2016;539(7630):560–4.
52. Silva R, Singh R, Sarker B, et al. Hydrogel matrices based on elastin and alginate for tissue engineering applications. *Int J Biol Macromol.* 2018;114:614–25.

53. Dutta SD, Patel DK, Lim KT. Functional cellulose-based hydrogels as extracellular matrices for tissue engineering. *J Biol Eng.* 2019;13:55.
54. Lannagan TRM, Lee YK, Wang T, et al. Genetic editing of colonic organoids provides a molecularly distinct and orthotopic preclinical model of serrated carcinogenesis. *Gut.* 2019;68(4):684–92.
55. Takeda H, Kataoka S, Nakayama M, et al. CRISPR-Cas9-mediated gene knockout in intestinal tumor organoids provides functional validation for colorectal cancer driver genes. *Proc Natl Acad Sci U S A.* 2019;*116*(31):15635–44.
56. Huch M, Dorrell C, Boj SF, et al. In vitro expansion of single Lgr5+ liver stem cells induced by Wnt-driven regeneration. *Nature.* 2013;494(7436):247–50.
57. Hunter BD, Chen YB, Jacobson CA. Allogeneic Stem Cell Transplantation and Chimeric Antigen Receptor (CAR) T-Cell Therapy for the Treatment of Non-Hodgkin Lymphoma. *Hematol Oncol Clin North Am.* 2019;33(4):687–705.
58. Schnalzger TE, de Groot MH, Zhang C, et al. 3D model for CAR-mediated cytotoxicity using patient-derived colorectal cancer organoids. *EMBO J.* 2019;38(12).
59. Michie J, Beavis PA, Freeman AJ, et al. Antagonism of IAPs Enhances CAR T-cell Efficacy. *Cancer Immunol Res.* 2019;7(2):183–92.
60. Chen J, Lau BT, Andor N, et al. Single-cell transcriptome analysis identifies distinct cell types and niche signaling in a primary gastric organoid model. *Sci Rep.* 2019;9(1):4536.
61. Pasch CA, Favreau PF, Yueh AE, et al. Patient-Derived Cancer Organoid Cultures to Predict Sensitivity to Chemotherapy and Radiation. *Clin Cancer Res.* 2019;25(17):5376–87.
62. Kong J. Tumor-Infiltrating lymphocyte function predicts response to neoadjuvant chemoradiotherapy in locally advanced rectal cancer. *JCO Precision oncology.* 2018;2:1–15.
63. Chen TW, Huang KC, Chiang SF, Chen WT, Ke TW, Chao KSC. Prognostic relevance of programmed cell death-ligand 1 expression and CD8+ TILs in rectal cancer patients before and after neoadjuvant chemoradiotherapy. *J Cancer Res Clin Oncol.* 2019;145(4):1043–53.
64. Cercek A, Lumish M, Sinopoli J, et al. PD-1 Blockade in Mismatch Repair-Deficient, Locally Advanced Rectal Cancer. *N Engl J Med.* 2022.
65. Thibodeau SN, Bren G, Schaid D. Microsatellite instability in cancer of the proximal colon. *Science.* 1993;260(5109):816–19.
66. Jenkins RW, Aref AR, Lizotte PH, et al. Ex Vivo Profiling of PD-1 Blockade Using Organotypic Tumor Spheroids. *Cancer Discov.* 2018;8(2):196–215.
67. Roerink SF, Sasaki N, Lee-Six H, et al. Intra-tumour diversification in colorectal cancer at the single-cell level. *Nature.* 2018;556(7702):457–62.
68. Fumagalli A, Drost J, Suijkerbuijk SJ, et al. Genetic dissection of colorectal cancer progression by orthotopic transplantation of engineered cancer organoids. *Proc Natl Acad Sci U S A.* 2017;114(12):E2357–E2364.
69. Takebe T, Wells JM. Organoids by design. *Science.* 2019;364(6444):956–59.
70. Workman MJ, Gleeson JP, Troisi EJ, et al. Enhanced utilization of induced pluripotent stem cell-derived human intestinal organoids using microengineered chips. *Cell Mol Gastroenterol Hepatol.* 2018;5(4):669–77 e662.
71. Skardal A, Murphy SV, Devarasetty M, et al. Multi-tissue interactions in an integrated three-tissue organ-on-a-chip platform. *Sci Rep.* 2017;7(1):8837.

15
Role of ctDNA in organ-preserving approaches to rectal cancer

Lauren O'Connell, Ben Creavin, and Desmond Winter

Cell-free DNA

Cell-free DNA (cfDNA) refers to circulating non-cell bound fragments of DNA. These may be derived from a variety of cell types, including those which have undergone malignant transformation. The phenomenon was first described in 1948 by Mandel and Metais; however, the significance of this finding did not become apparent until 1977, when it was found that the serum concentration of cfDNA was substantially higher in cancer patients than healthy controls.[1,2]

Although first detected in blood, cfDNA is also present in other bodily fluids including urine, cerebrospinal fluid, and saliva.[3,4] It has a short half-life of 16 minutes to several hours.[5] The presence of cfDNA is a normal occurrence at low concentrations in healthy individuals, as nucleoprotein complexes are released by human leukocytes and haematopoietic cells.[6] Increased concentrations of cfDNA are also seen in a number of physiological and pathological conditions, including exercise, pregnancy, infarction, sepsis, trauma, and transplant recipients.[7–13] In pregnancy, both maternal and foetal cfDNA can be detected in maternal serum, facilitating prenatal diagnosis of foetal genetic abnormalities.[14] cfDNA may also have utility as a prognostic biomarker in sepsis.[13]

Circulating tumour DNA

However, the greatest application of cfDNA to date has undoubtedly been in the field of oncology. Circulating tumour DNA (ctDNA) refers specifically to the fraction of cell-free DNA derived from malignant cells. The quantity of ctDNA released varies according to tumour type. ctDNA derived from colorectal, gastro-oesophageal, pancreatic, and breast tumours is commonly detectable in serum in early localized disease, while it remains undetectable in over 50% of advanced thyroid and brain malignancies.[5] Quantity of ctDNA also correlates with disease burden, with higher volumes seen in advanced and metastatic disease.[5,15,16]

Multiple theories have been advanced as to the mechanism by which cfDNA occurs. The primary theories are that it is a byproduct of cellular apoptosis and necrosis. Other theories include that it arises from the lysis of circulating tumour cells (CTCs). However, cfDNA is commonly detectable in serum in the absence of CTCs; further, the usual concentration of CTCs is too low to produce the quantity of cfDNA normally found in serum.[5] Active secretion of nucleic acids by the primary tumour has also been proposed, with a transfection-like process occurring in healthy cells and thus contributing to malignant transformation. This theory is referred to as 'genometastasis'. Although the genometastasis theory is not as well supported as the others, some evidence does exist that ctDNA can seed and induce malignant transformation of healthy tissues.[17]

However, the theories relating to apoptosis and necrosis currently appear most plausible. The cfDNA that occurs in healthy individuals and physiological conditions such as pregnancy is attributed to the former, as the fragment lengths produced are uniform (<185 bp) and are known to result from the DNA cleavage that occurs in apoptosis.[18] By contrast, longer (>250 bp) and more variable fragment lengths are produced in necrotic cell death. These longer fragments contain tumour-specific sequences and so can be distinguished as arising from malignant cells.[6,19]

As described earlier, the process of apoptosis produces short fragments of <185 bp, while ctDNA arising from necrosis produces longer fragments (>250 bp). This disparity in fragment length is utilized in the DNA integrity index (DII). This calculates the ratio of short to long fragments to determine what proportion of cfDNA detected is a result of necrosis and therefore likely to be tumour-derived.[20,21] Incorporating the DII into diagnostic algorithms has been shown to improve the sensitivity and specificity over quantitative measurement of cfDNA alone for the diagnosis of malignancy.[5] More sophisticated methods than simple quantification of ctDNA also exist. Assessment of promoter hypermethylation, microsatellite instability, chromosomal rearrangements, copy number variations, and single-nucleotide polymorphisms (SNPs) can be performed from a 'liquid biopsy' of ctDNA alone.[5,22,23]

Detection of ctDNA

Dependent on tumour stage and type, ctDNA can comprise a highly variable proportion of the total cfDNA. In metastatic disease, it can represent up to 50% while in early stage cancers as little as 0.01%.[24–26] Thus, methods of ctDNA detection, particularly for the purpose of early diagnosis or detection in a screening population, must be highly sensitive and reproducible.

Current methods being utilized for ctDNA detection and analysis are differentiated into targeted and untargeted approaches. Targeted approaches detect specific, predetermined molecular aberrations. These methods have the capacity to overcome many of the difficulties associated with ctDNA detection, including small sample volumes, short DNA fragment length, and low diagnostic allele frequency. Non-targeted methods do not require prior knowledge of tumour-specific molecular alterations and utilize whole-genome or whole-exome sequencing. While non-targeted methods are useful for detecting novel tumour-specific mutations and epigenetic modifications, they are relatively high-cost and poorer at detecting rare allele variants than targeted methods. Thus, targeted methods are more frequently utilized for clinical applications.

Digital polymerized chain reaction (PCR)

Digital PCR methods are targeted methods, which broadly include droplet digital PCR (ddPCR) and beads, emulsion, amplification, and magnetics (BEAMing). These methods have a particularly low limit of detection of mutant alleles, with the limit of detection for ddPCR and BEAMing 0.001% and 0.01%, respectively. They have a high sensitivity and specificity, but only moderate cost relative to other methods and are not technically difficult to perform. However, the genes detected need to be predetermined by the operator and only a limited number of genes can be interrogated at a time.[24,,27,28] Allele-specific quantitative PCR is another highly sensitive targeted method with similar cost and analysis considerations as ddPCR and BEAMing.[29]

Next-generation sequencing

Next-generation sequencing (NGS) methods can be used to perform whole-genome analysis, or applied to targeted gene panels. Methods utilized in targeted gene panels include amplicon-based sequencing and hybridization capture methods. As with digital PCR, the panels are based on previously known genes, but based on larger target regions than is possible with digital PCR. They therefore allow simultaneous interrogation of multiple gene loci. However, larger DNA quantities are required than for digital PCR, and the process is slower. The sensitivity of these methods is variable. Amplicon-based methods have a limit of detection of 0.1–2%, while hybridization capture methods have a limit of detection approaching digital PCR methods of 0.01%. They are, however, less sensitive than digital PCR for detection of rare allele variants. The volume of data produced is also substantially larger and requires bioinformatic assistance for analysis. They are also expensive, costing >$900 per panel. However, amplicon-based and hybridization capture methods remain more sensitive and cheaper than whole-genome or whole-exome sequencing.[30,31]

Genome-wide analysis

Genome-wide analysis employs either whole-genome or whole-exome sequencing methods. As it only sequences exons rather than both exons and non-coding DNA, whole-exome sequencing is less expensive and produces a lower volume of data than whole-genome sequencing. These methods are superior at mapping tumour heterogeneity as they can detect tumour-specific copy number variations, chromosomal rearrangements, and other structural changes which are not detectable by targeted methods. However, they are the most expensive of all the methods, and the sensitivity and specificity are dependent on allele frequency and abundance of the sequence.[23,31,32]

Clinical applications of ctDNA with respect to LARC

Prediction of response to naCRT and pretreatment risk stratification

Response to chemoradiotherapy is an important prognostic indicator in rectal cancer.[33] A pCR to nCRT is associated with good long-term outcomes, including improved 5-year disease-free survival.[34] Radical surgery, although providing excellent oncologic outcomes, nonetheless carries risks of short-term morbidity and long-term functional impairment.[35,36]

A biomarker accurately predicting response to nCRT would allow pretreatment stratification of patients with LARC. Those with a high likelihood of pCR would thus avoid unnecessary surgery. In those predicted to have a less favourable response, neoadjuvant treatment could be intensified with systemic chemotherapy. In patients where nCRT is predicted to be of negligible impact, this would permit avoidance of unnecessary treatment-related toxicity.

Some factors for predicting response already exist, such as pretreatment CEA levels, which are an independent prognostic marker for pCR. However, as a biomarker CEA suffers from limited sensitivity and specificity.[37–39] A number of studies have investigated the role of ctDNA as a predictor of response to nCRT.[40–46] Only one study demonstrated a significant correlation between baseline ctDNA concentrations and response to nCRT. Sun observed in a small study of 34 patients that good responders had significantly higher pretreatment levels of 400bp fragments and a significantly higher DII.[41] However, no significant association in baseline ctDNA levels with nCRT response was demonstrated in the other six studies.

Advantages of ctDNA as a biomarker include that it can provide for superior mapping of tumour heterogeneity and mutational landscape over tissue diagnosis. The latter is necessarily a spatially limited sample and represents only a single timepoint.[47,48] This is particularly relevant given that many studies have suggested that molecular factors play a role in tumour responsiveness, with KRAS mutations associated with resistance to nCRT.[49,50] One series of 148 patients demonstrated a lower rate of pCR in tumours with mutant KRAS compared to wild-type ($p = 0.006$).[49] Other factors such as EGFR expression pattern and presence of promoter hypermethylation may also have value in predicting response to treatment.[51,52] KRAS status can be reliably determined from blood-derived ctDNA with a specificity of 98–100% and concordance with tissue of 82%.[5,6,24,25] Epigenetic changes can also be readily detected using either digital PCR or NGS methods and correlate well with tissue.[6,51]

Thus, measurement of baseline concentrations of ctDNA alone does not appear to be a useful predictor of response to nCRT in LARC. However, ctDNA may play a useful role in determining the molecular profile of the tumour.

Guidance of treatment paradigms

As described earlier, a cohort of patients with LARC exists with factors that predict a poor response to nCRT. In addition, definitive chemoradiotherapy is being increasingly advanced as a novel treatment option in clinical trials.[53,54] To boost efficacy in these instances, the neoadjuvant treatment paradigm may be altered to incorporate elements usually reserved for adjuvant treatment. This includes systemic therapy but also targeted anti-EGFR therapies such as cetuximab and panitumumab. ctDNA is highly reliable for the detection of KRAS status and demonstrates strong concordance with tissue. Mutations also implicated in EGFR resistance, such as *PTEN*, *NRAS*, and *BRAF V600E* can also be elucidated from ctDNA blood samples with a high degree of accuracy; concordance between tissue and blood-derived ctDNA BRAF mutation detection was 100% in two studies by Thierry and Taly.[24,25] Therefore, ctDNA can play a useful role in determining response to targeted therapies.

In addition, clonal evolution and emerging treatment resistance can be tracked in a dynamic fashion, as multiple serial ctDNA samples can be acquired during treatment.[26,55] Further, ctDNA detection of declining EGFR resistance once treatment is withdrawn has been demonstrated, permitting successful re-challenge with anti-EGFR agents.[56]

Detection of minimal residual disease and early detection of recurrence

Detection of the proportion of patients who have a true pCR after nCRT versus those who harbour residual disease represents an ongoing challenge. A cCR based on clinical examination, endoscopic, and radiological findings is currently used as a surrogate marker for pCR. The ACCORD 12/PRODIGE 2 trial found a significant association between cCR response and ypT0 and ypN0 (73% and 92%, respectively, $p < 0.001$) pathological specimens. However, mucosal abnormalities at endoscopy and mixed signal intensity due to fibrotic changes on MRI can produce discrepancies in the endoscopic and MRI radiological evaluation of response compared to that found on pathological examination.[57,58] Thus, a need exists for a biomarker which can assist in discriminating between minimal residual disease (MRD) and pCR in patients post-nCRT, and can predict early recurrence in those undergoing a strategy of watchful waiting.

Initial tumour burden as estimated by RECIST criteria (Response Evaluation Criteria in Solid Tumors) is associated with increased levels of ctDNA, with tumour volume in particular strongly correlated to ctDNA concentration.[16,19,59] While previously described studies evaluating the role of ctDNA as a predictor of treatment response in LARC do not conclusively demonstrate a predictive role for baseline ctDNA levels, assessment of ctDNA levels post-delivery of nCRT shows substantially more promise.

An early study by Zitt in 2008 analysed ctDNA levels in LARC pre- and post-nCRT and post-total mesorectal excision (TME). There was no significant difference in median ctDNA levels prior to or post-nCRT. However, dynamic changes in ctDNA levels in individuals over the course of treatment were significantly predictive of response, with decreased ctDNA levels seen in responders (mean 2.2 ng/ml) and increased levels seen in non-responders (mean 5.1 ng/ml, $p < 0.006$). Another study by Agostini in 2011, which assessed the DII pre- and post-nCRT demonstrated similar findings, with the integrity index significantly lower post-nCRT in responders than in non-responders ($p < 0.0009$) but not discriminatory at baseline.[40] In both studies response to treatment was confirmed at histology.

A small case series by Carpinetti of four patients assessed ctDNA levels using tumour-specific chromosomal rearrangements pre- and post-nCRT and during follow-up. ctDNA was undetectable in three of the four patients post-treatment, although only one had a pCR with the others demonstrating a partial response.[42] Thus, although lacking sufficient sensitivity to accurately detect MRD post-nCRT, the study did suggest a potentially useful role for ctDNA in early detection of recurrence, as elevated ctDNA levels were present in the two patients who ultimately developed distant metastases. Interestingly, in one patient, the elevated ctDNA levels preceded radiological evidence of relapse by four months.

A more recent study published by Tie in 2019 (n = 159) found no difference in three-year recurrence-free survival (RFS) for those with detectable ctDNA pretreatment. However, detectable ctDNA after either surgery or nCRT was an independent predictor of increased risk of recurrence, with a 33% three-year RFS in this cohort versus 87% for those with undetectable ctDNA.[45] In this study, detectable ctDNA post-treatment had superior prognostic value to CEA for the prediction of recurrence.

A similar Danish study of 123 rectal cancer patients demonstrated that baseline ctDNA levels above the 75th percentile were associated with significantly higher rates of local and distant recurrence, shorter time to recurrence (HR 2.48, $p = 0.007$) and poorer disease-free survival (HR 2.43, $p = 0.015$) compared to those with lower rates of ctDNA.[44]

Conclusion

Thus, the incorporation of ctDNA into a combined predictive model along with established factors such as CEA could feasibly refine the therapeutic strategy in LARC, maximizing the delivery of organ-preserving approaches to eligible patients and expediting surgery for non-responders. It also demonstrates promise as a tool for early detection of recurrence in those patients undergoing watchful waiting.

Due to techniques such as digital PCR and NGS, it is also likely to play a valuable role in profiling the heterogeneous mutational landscape of rectal cancer. This will assist in risk stratification, prediction of response to chemoradiotherapy and eligibility for biological therapies.

References

1. Mandel P, Metais P. [Not Available]. *C R Seances Soc Biol Fil.* 1948;142(3–4):241–3.
2. Leon SA, Shapiro B, Sklaroff DM, Yaros MJ. Free DNA in the serum of cancer patients and the effect of therapy. *Cancer Res.* 1977;37(3):646–50.
3. De Mattos-Arruda L, Mayor R, Ng CKY, et al. Cerebrospinal fluid-derived circulating tumour DNA better represents the genomic alterations of brain tumours than plasma. *Nat Commun.* 2015;6:8839.
4. Wang Y, Springer S, Mulvey CL, et al. Detection of somatic mutations and HPV in the saliva and plasma of patients with head and neck squamous cell carcinomas. *Sci Transl Med.* 2015;7(293):293ra104.
5. Bettegowda C, Sausen M, Leary RJ, et al. Detection of circulating tumor DNA in early- and late-stage human malignancies. *Sci Transl Med.* 2014;6(224):224ra24.
6. Petit J, Carroll G, Gould T, Pockney P, Dun M, Scott RJ. Cell-free DNA as a diagnostic blood-based biomarker for colorectal cancer: a systematic review. *J Surg Res.* 2019;236:184–97.
7. Schütz E, Fischer A, Beck J, et al. Graft-derived cell-free DNA, a noninvasive early rejection and graft damage marker in liver transplantation: a prospective, observational, multicenter cohort study. *PLoS Med.* 2017;14(4):e1002286.
8. Jing R, Cui M, Wang H, Ju S. Cell-free DNA: characteristics, detection and its applications in myocardial infarction. *Curr Pharm Des.* 2013;19(28):5135–45.
9. Bianchi DW, Chiu RWK. Sequencing of circulating cell-free DNA during pregnancy. *N Engl J Med.* 2018;379(5):464–73.
10. Gögenur M, Burcharth J, Gögenur I. The role of total cell-free DNA in predicting outcomes among trauma patients in the intensive care unit: a systematic review. *Crit Care.* 2017;21(1):14.
11. Vittori LN, Tarozzi A, Latessa PM. Circulating cell-free DNA in physical activities. *Methods Mol Biol.* 2019;1909:183–97.
12. Hampson P, Dinsdale RJ, Wearn CM, et al. Neutrophil dysfunction, immature granulocytes, and cell-free DNA are early biomarkers of sepsis in burn-injured patients: a prospective observational cohort study. *Ann Surg.* 2017;265(6):1241–9.
13. Hawkins RB, Stortz JA, Holden DC, et al. Persistently increased cell-free DNA concentrations only modestly contribute to outcome and host response in sepsis survivors with chronic critical illness. *Surgery.* 2020;167(3):646–52.

14. Gil MM, Accurti V, Santacruz B, Plana MN, Nicolaides KH. Analysis of cell-free DNA in maternal blood in screening for aneuploidies: updated meta-analysis. *Ultrasound Obstet Gynecol.* 2017;50(3):302–14.
15. Fiala C, Diamandis EP. Utility of circulating tumor DNA in cancer diagnostics with emphasis on early detection. *BMC Med.* 2018;16(1):166.
16. Tie J, Kinde I, Wang Y, et al. Circulating tumor DNA as an early marker of therapeutic response in patients with metastatic colorectal cancer. *Ann Oncol.* 2015;26(8):1715–22.
17. Garcia-Olmo DC, Dominguez C, Garcia-Arranz M, JM, et al. Cell-free nucleic acids circulating in the plasma of colorectal cancer patients induce the oncogenic transformation of susceptible cultured cells. *Cancer Res.* 2010;70:560–7.
18. Giacona MB, Ruben GC, Iczkowski KA, Roos TB, Porter DM, Sorenson GD. Cell-free DNA in human blood plasma. *Pancreas.* 1998;17:89–97.
19. Osumi H, Shinozaki E, Takeda Y, et al. Clinical relevance of circulating tumor DNA assessed through deep sequencing in patients with metastatic colorectal cancer. *Cancer Med.* 2019;8(1):408–17.
20. Leszinski G, Lehner J, Gezer U, Holdenrieder S. Increased DNA integrity in colorectal cancer. *In Vivo.* 2014;28(3):299–303.
21. Lehner J, Stötzer OJ, Fersching D, Nagel D, Holdenrieder S. Circulating plasma DNA and DNA integrity in breast cancer patients undergoing neoadjuvant chemotherapy. *Clin Chim Acta.* 2013;425:206–11.
22. Moati E, Taly V, Didelot A, et al. Role of circulating tumor DNA in the management of patients with colorectal cancer. *Clin Res Hepatol Gastroenterol.* 2018;42(5):396–402.
23. Osumi H, Shinozaki E, Yamaguchi K, Zembutsu H. Clinical utility of circulating tumor DNA for colorectal cancer. *Cancer Sci.* 2019;110(4):1148–55.
24. Taly V, Pekin D, Benhaim L, et al. Multiplex picodroplet digital PCR to detect KRAS mutations in circulating DNA from the plasma of colorectal cancer patients. *Clin Chem.* 2013;59(12):1722–31.
25. Thierry AR, Mouliere F, El Messaoudi S, et al. Clinical validation of the detection of KRAS and BRAF mutations from circulating tumor DNA. *Nat Med.* 2014;20(4):430–5.
26. Misale S, Yaeger R, Hobor S, et al. Emergence of KRAS mutations and acquired resistance to anti-EGFR therapy in colorectal cancer. *Nature.* 2012;486(7404):532–6.
27. Diehl F, Li M, He Y, Kinzler KW, Vogelstein B, Dressman D. BEAMing: single-molecule PCR on microparticles in water-in-oil emulsions. *Nat Methods.* 2006;3(7):551–9.
28. Day E, Dear PH, McCaughan F. Digital PCR strategies in the development and analysis of molecular biomarkers for personalized medicine. *Methods.* 2013;59(1):101–7.
29. Mouliere F, El Messaoudi S, Pang D, Dritschilo A, Thierry AR. Multi-marker analysis of circulating cell-free DNA toward personalized medicine for colorectal cancer. *Mol Oncol.* 2014;8(5):927–41.
30. Lanman RB, Mortimer SA, Zill OA, et al. Analytical and clinical validation of a digital sequencing panel for quantitative, highly accurate evaluation of cell-free circulating tumor DNA. *PLoS One.* 2015;10(10):e0140712.
31. Chen M, Zhao H. Next-generation sequencing in liquid biopsy: cancer screening and early detection. *Hum Genomics.* 2019;13(1):34.
32. Manier S, Park J, Capelletti M, et al. Whole-exome sequencing of cell-free DNA and circulating tumor cells in multiple myeloma. *Nat Commun.* 2018;9(1):1691.
33. Molinari C, Matteucci F, Caroli P, Passardi A. Biomarkers and molecular imaging as predictors of response to neoadjuvant chemoradiotherapy in patients with locally advanced rectal cancer. *Clin Colorectal Cancer.* 2015;14(4):227–38.

34. Maas M, Nelemans PJ, Valentini V, et al. Long-term outcome in patients with a pathological complete response after chemoradiation for rectal cancer: a pooled analysis of individual patient data. *Lancet Oncol.* 2010;11(9):835–44.
35. Ozgen Z, Ozden S, Atasoy BM, Ozyurt H, Gencosmanoglu R, Imeryuz N. Long-term effects of neoadjuvant chemoradiotherapy followed by sphincter-preserving resection on anal sphincter function in relation to quality of life among locally advanced rectal cancer patients: a cross-sectional analysis. *Radiat Oncol.* 2015;10:168.
36. van Gijn W, Marijnen CAM, Nagtegaal ID, et al. Preoperative radiotherapy combined with total mesorectal excision for resectable rectal cancer: 12-year follow-up of the multicentre, randomised controlled TME trial. *Lancet Oncol.* 2011;12(6):575–82.
37. Park JW, Lim S-B, Kim DY, et al. Carcinoembryonic antigen as a predictor of pathologic response and a prognostic factor in locally advanced rectal cancer patients treated with preoperative chemoradiotherapy and surgery. *Int J Radiat Oncol Biol Physics.* 2009;74(3):810–17.
38. Restivo A, Zorcolo L, Cocco IMF, et al. Elevated CEA levels and low distance of the tumor from the anal verge are predictors of incomplete response to chemoradiation in patients with rectal cancer. *Ann Surg Oncol.* 2013;20(3):864–71.
39. Wallin U, Rothenberger D, Lowry A, Luepker R, Mellgren A. CEA—a predictor for pathologic complete response after neoadjuvant therapy for rectal cancer. *Dis Colon Rectum.* 2013;56(7):859–68.
40. Agostini M, Pucciarelli S, Enzo MV, et al. Circulating cell-free DNA: a promising marker of pathologic tumor response in rectal cancer patients receiving preoperative chemoradiotherapy. *Ann Surg Oncol.* 2011;18(9):2461–8.
41. Sun W, Sun Y, Zhu M, et al. The role of plasma cell-free DNA detection in predicting preoperative chemoradiotherapy response in rectal cancer patients. *Oncol Rep.* 2014;31(3):1466–72.
42. Carpinetti P, Donnard E, Bettoni F, et al. The use of personalized biomarkers and liquid biopsies to monitor treatment response and disease recurrence in locally advanced rectal cancer after neoadjuvant chemoradiation. *Oncotarget.* 2015;6(35):38360–71.
43. Zitt M, Müller HM, Rochel M, et al. Circulating cell-free DNA in plasma of locally advanced rectal cancer patients undergoing preoperative chemoradiation: a potential diagnostic tool for therapy monitoring. *Dis Markers.* 2008;25:159–65.
44. Schou JV, Larsen FO, Sørensen BS, et al. Circulating cell-free DNA as predictor of treatment failure after neoadjuvant chemo-radiotherapy before surgery in patients with locally advanced rectal cancer. *Ann Oncol.* 2018;29(3):610–15.
45. Tie J, Cohen JD, Wang Y, et al. Serial circulating tumour DNA analysis during multimodality treatment of locally advanced rectal cancer: a prospective biomarker study. *Gut.* 2019;68(4):663–71.
46. Zhou J, Lin G, Gong Y, et al. Serial ctDNA analysis as a real-time indicator of neoadjuvant chemoradiotherapy in rectal cancer. *J Clin Orthod.* 2019;37(15_suppl):3569.
47. Thierry AR, El Messaoudi S, Mollevi C, et al. Clinical utility of circulating DNA analysis for rapid detection of actionable mutations to select metastatic colorectal patients for anti-EGFR treatment. *Ann Oncol.* 2017;28(9):2149–59.
48. Siravegna G, Marsoni S, Siena S, Bardelli A. Integrating liquid biopsies into the management of cancer. *Nat Rev Clin Oncol.* 2017;14(9):531–48.
49. Duldulao MP, Lee W, Nelson RA, et al. Mutations in specific codons of the KRAS oncogene are associated with variable resistance to neoadjuvant chemoradiation therapy in patients with rectal adenocarcinoma. *Ann Surg Oncol.* 2013;20(7):2166–71.

50. Garcia-Aguilar J, Chen Z, Smith DD, et al. Identification of a biomarker profile associated with resistance to neoadjuvant chemoradiation therapy in rectal cancer. *Ann Surg.* 2011;254(3):486–92; discussion 492–3.
51. Shalaby SM, El-Shal AS, Abdelaziz LA, Abd-Elbary E, Khairy MM. Promoter methylation and expression of DNA repair genes MGMT and ERCC1 in tissue and blood of rectal cancer patients. *Gene.* 2018;644:66–73.
52. Chen C-T, Tufts L, Aggarwal P, Heller F, Weiser MR. Detection of methylated BCAT1 and IKZF1 in stage II/III rectal cancer receiving chemoradiation. *J Clin Orthod.* 2019;37(4_suppl):602.
53. Yoo RN, Kim HJ. Total neoadjuvant therapy in locally advanced rectal cancer: Role of systemic chemotherapy. *Ann Gastroenterol Surg.* 2019;3(4):356–67.
54. Franke AJ, Parekh H, Starr JS, Tan SA, Iqbal A, George TJ Jr. Total neoadjuvant therapy: a shifting paradigm in locally advanced rectal cancer management. *Clin Colorectal Cancer.* 2018;17(1):1–12.
55. Siravegna G, Mussolin B, Buscarino M, et al. Clonal evolution and resistance to EGFR blockade in the blood of colorectal cancer patients. *Nat Med.* 2015;21(7):827.
56. Parseghian CM, Loree JM, Morris VK, et al. Anti-EGFR-resistant clones decay exponentially after progression: implications for anti-EGFR re-challenge. *Ann Oncol.* 2019;30(2):243–9.
57. van der Sande ME, Beets GL, Hupkens BJ, et al. Response assessment after (chemo)radiotherapy for rectal cancer: why are we missing complete responses with MRI and endoscopy? *Eur J Surg Oncol.* 2019;45(6):1011–17.
58. Liu S, Zhong G-X, Zhou W-X, et al. Can endorectal ultrasound, MRI, and mucosa integrity accurately predict the complete response for mid-low rectal cancer after preoperative chemoradiation? A prospective observational study from a single medical center. *Dis Colon Rectum.* 2018;61(8):903–10.
59. Wang J-Y, Hsieh J-S, Chang M-Y, et al. Molecular detection of APC, K- ras, and p53 mutations in the serum of colorectal cancer patients as circulating biomarkers. *World J Surg.* 2004;28(7):721–6.

16

Predicting pathological response to neoadjuvant chemoradiotherapy in locally advanced rectal cancer

Alexandra Zaborowski, Ben Creavin, and Kieran Sheahan

Clinical factors

Studies have identified lower pretreatment cT stage, cN stage, and American Joint Committee on Cancer (AJCC) cTNM stage as predictive factors associated with increased likelihood of pathological complete response (pCR).[1,2] A retrospective analysis of 391 patients observed higher rates of pCR among patients with noncircumferential tumours (OR, 3.214, p = 0.007), non-macroscopic ulceration (OR, 6.702, p = 0.002), and low pretreatment CEA level (OR, 2.656, p = 0.004).[3] Patel et al. investigated the relationship between distance to anal verge and pCR among 827 patients and found that patients with low tumours (<4 cm) and higher tumours (>8 cm), were less likely to have a pCR (p = 0.002).[4]

Numerous studies have observed improved tumour regression among patients with low pretreatment CEA levels. A retrospective analysis of 469 patients undergoing conventional 5-FU-based neoadjuvant CRT found that low pretreatment CEA was significantly associated with pCR (p = 0.008).[5] A smaller study by Huh et al. also found low pretreatment carcinoembryonic antigen (CEA) level to be an independent predictor of pCR (OR, 2.656, p = 0.004).[3] Post-treatment CEA level appears to represent a proxy measure for pathological response. One of the largest studies categorized 659 patients into two groups according to post-treatment serum CEA level: low CEA (<5 ng/ml) and high CEA (≥ 5 ng/ml), and found that a high post-CRT level was significantly associated with ypTNM stage, ypT stage, and poor tumour regression.[6] Similarly, other series have also identified low post-treatment CEA level as a favourable predictor of pathological response.[7,8]

Pathological factors

Mismatch repair status

Approximately 15% of colorectal cancers (CRCs) develop via defective DNA mismatch repair (MMR), resulting in microsatellite instability.[9] This defect may be caused by sporadic events (e.g. epigenetic silencing of the MLH1 gene) or by constitutive mutations in one of the MMR genes—the most common of which are MLH1, MSH2, MSH6, and PMS2—resulting in the most common hereditary cancer syndrome (Lynch syndrome).[10] The National Comprehensive Cancer Network (NCCN) guidelines now recommend routine analysis of MMR status for all patients with CRC, with subsequent germline testing performed as needed.[11]

Dichotomization of CRC into pMMR and dMMR has important prognostic and therapeutic implications. Clinical data suggest that dMMR tumours are less likely to metastasize to lymph nodes and distant organs, and are associated with better stage-specific survival.[12] Interestingly, the 'protective' effect of dMMR may be lost in lymph node positive disease, and disease-specific survival was comparable to that of pMMR tumours of the same stage in a single institutional study.[13] The benefit of 5-fluorouracil-based chemotherapy is controversial in dMMR, with some studies suggesting relative resistance.[14,15]

Pathological response to conventional neoadjuvant fluoropyrimidine-based chemoradiotherapy among patients with dMMR rectal cancer remains undefined, with available data conflicting. A single-centre retrospective study reported a pCR rate of 27.6% among 30 patients, suggesting a greater response.[16] In contrast, a large registry-based study of 5,086 patients with microsatellite instability (MSI) rectal cancer found a pCR rate of 5.9% for MSI-positive (MSI+) and 8.9% for MSI-negative (MSI-), $p = 0.01$.[17] On multivariable analysis, MSI+ cases were significantly associated with a reduced pCR rate (OR 0.65).

Conventional neoadjuvant therapy is currently the standard of care for LARC regardless of MMR status. The influence of MMR status on radiosensitivity, and whether MMR status should guide therapeutic decision-making is unclear. Ionizing radiation exerts direct genotoxic effects on tumour cell DNA, culminating in apoptosis. Accumulating evidence suggests that MMR proteins play a direct and indirect role in this DNA damage response, conferring greater sensitivity to IR.[18,19] The mechanism of MMR-related sensitivity appears to depend on the dose of radiotherapy administered. Acute high-dose IR is associated with radiosensitivity in MMR deficiency, while low-dose IR is associated with radiosensitivity in MMR-proficiency.

Mucinous histology

Mucinous tumours are defined as lesions in which >50% of the tumour volume consists of pools of extracellular mucin and account for approximately 5–15% of CRC.[20]

The mucinous subtype represents a negative prognostic indicator. It is associated with poorer response to neoadjuvant CRT, higher positive margins, and worse survival compared to non-mucinous tumours.[21,22] Despite a reliable diagnosis of mucinous differentiation on pretreatment biopsies and T2-weighted MRI, it is not currently used as a biomarker of response to neoadjuvant therapy.[23]

The molecular mechanisms underlying the apparent radioresistance of mucinous tumours are poorly understood. Alternative oncogenic mutations and pathways have been postulated to play a role.[24] A meta-analysis found mucinous histology was positively associated with *BRAF* mutations (OR 3.49), MSI (OR 3.98), CIMP-high status (OR 3.56), and negatively associated with altered p53 expression (OR 0.46).[25] Less apoptotic activity has also been observed in mucinous tumours,[26] which may in part account for the poor response to CRT as apoptosis represents a known mechanism by which radiotherapy exerts its anti-tumour effect.[27]

Mucinous tumours have also been associated with relative chemoresistance and reduced responsiveness to 5-FU-based chemotherapeutic regimes.[28,29] It is possible that decreased pathological response rates to neoadjuvant CRT among the mucinous subtype may also in part be related to reduced efficacy of the radiosensitizing chemotherapy component of the neoadjuvant protocol. Regimes such as XELOX or FOLFIRI, alone or in combination with targeted therapies may be more effective. These agents have largely been studied in metastatic CRC only, and their role in the neoadjuvant setting for LARC is unknown.

Tumour budding

Tumour budding is a histopathological feature of epithelial cancers whereby isolated tumour cells or clusters of fewer than five cells detach from the invasive margin and migrate into the surrounding stroma.[30] Present in 20–40% of CRC, it is considered a morphological manifestation of epithelial-mesenchymal transition and represents a negative prognostic indicator in CRC.[31] A meta-analysis including 7,821 patients found tumour budding was associated with an increased likelihood of lymph node positivity (OR 4.94), disease recurrence (OR 5.50), and cancer-related mortality at 5 years (OR 4.51).[31,32]

Several studies have evaluated the prognostic value of tumour budding in rectal cancer prior to neoadjuvant radio(chemo)therapy.[33,34] Intratumoural budding in pretreatment biopsies was significantly associated with unfavourable prognostic factors in the resected tumour specimen, including higher ypT stage, residual lymph node involvement, poor differentiation, and lymphovascular invasion. Furthermore, budding was strongly predictive of a poor pathological response to neoadjuvant CRT.

The biomolecular mechanisms underpinning the impact of tumour budding on pathological response are unclear. It has been postulated that the immune system may play a contributory role as tumour budding has been infrequently encountered in patients with robust peri-tumoural CD8+ T-cell infiltration.[35] The combination of tumour cell 'stemness' and a poor immune response may in part account for the relative radioresistance observed in patients exhibiting tumour budding.

Molecular factors

KRAS status

The V-Ki-ras2 Kirsten rat sarcoma viral oncogene (KRAS), an important component of the epidermal growth factor receptor (EGFR) pathway, is implicated in 30–40% of CRCs. KRAS status has been incorporated into treatment algorithms as a predictor of poor response to anti-EGFR monoclonal antibodies such as cetuximab and panitumumab in metastatic CRC.[36,37] Its role as a predictive biomarker in rectal cancer remains equivocal, and the data are conflicting. Several studies found that KRAS mutation status does not influence pathological response to preoperative CRT.[38,39] In contrast, Chow et al. observed that KRAS mutation was independently associated with a lower pCR rate among 229 patients.[40] Notably the neoadjuvant regime in this study included induction or consolidation FOLFOX. Mutational location has been postulated as playing a role in response. Patients with KRAS codon 13 mutations are less likely to achieve a pCR compared to those with mutations at codon 12.[41,42]

p53 status

Mutations in the p53 tumour suppressor gene (TSG) occur in 40–50% of CRCs. Data on the role of p53 status as a biomarker to predict response to neoadjuvant CRT in rectal cancer are inconsistent. Although several studies have reported no association between p53 status and response,[43,44] a meta-analysis of 30 studies including 1,830 patients suggested that wild-type form of p53 status was predictive of response.[45]

DNA methylation

Aberrant DNA methylation of cytosine-phosphate-guanine (CpG) islands, in particular the CpG island methylator phenotype (CIMP), occurs in approximately 2–10% of rectal cancers.[46,47] Clinicopathological features of CIMP-high tumours include a predilection for mucinous differentiation and BRAF mutations, while CIMP-low tumours are associated with KRAS mutations.[48]

The predictive value of DNA methylation patterns in response to neoadjuvant therapy for rectal cancer remains under investigation. Sun et al. observed higher rates of DNA repair enzyme O6-methylguanine-DNA methyltransferase (MGMT) promoter methylation among patients with a good response to neoadjuvant therapy compared to those with a poor response (88.9 vs. 50%, p = 0.04).[4]. Similarly, Molinari et al. characterized the methylation profiles of pretreatment biopsies in 77 patients and found hypermethylation of the TIMP3 tumour suppressor gene appeared to be associated with improved pathological response to neoadjuvant CRT.[50] Analysis of 23 other TSGs, however, identified no correlation between methylation status and response, suggesting that TIMP3 methylation status is not the principal biomarker of chemoradio-sensitivity. In contrast, Jo et al. found no correlation between CIMP status and tumour regression among 150 patients treated with neoadjuvant CRT.

Gene expression profiling

Several studies have used gene expression profiling in a bid to predict response to neoadjuvant CRT in rectal cancer. Gantt et al. identified a unique genetic signature associated with chemoradiation-resistant disease.[51] Total tumour mRNA was extracted from the pretreatment biopsies of 33 patients, and gene expression levels were measured using microarray analysis. An 812-gene signature was identified separating non-responders from responders, with a sensitivity and specificity of 100%. Using a bioinformatic approach, Gim et al. developed and validated a three-class classification model predicting minimal, moderate, or complete response to neoadjuvant CRT by analysing the gene expression profiles of 77 pretreatment biopsies.[52] Guo et al. found that genes associated with pathways involved in DNA replication, cell cycle, and DNA repair were upregulated in responders while genes associated with drug and protein metabolism were enriched in non-responders.[53] Although promising, gene expression profiling has yet to translate into routine clinical practice.

Single-nucleotide polymorphisms (SNPs)

Advances in large-scale genotyping have enabled the investigation of germline genetic markers, such as single-nucleotide polymorphisms (SNPs), in predicting pathological response to neoadjuvant CRT. SNPs within genes influence the expression or function of corresponding proteins and are thought to contribute to the variation in drug response observed among individuals. Thymidylate synthase is an important enzyme involved in DNA synthesis and is the primary target of 5-FU. Several studies have identified specific genetic polymorphisms in the thymidylate synthase (TYMS) gene associated with 5-FU-based chemoradio-sensitivity.[54,55]

Ho-Pun-Cheung et al. evaluated the predictive value of 128 SNPs distributed over 76 genes in 71 patients treated with neoadjuvant CRT, and found that SNPs superoxide dismutase 2 (SOD2) rs4880 (p = 0.005) and interleukin-13 rs1800925 (p = 0.0008) were significantly associated with tumour response.[56] Similarly, genome-wide screening of 43 patients identified 9 SNPs associated with CRT response.[57] Two CRT-sensitive SNPs, CORO2A rs1985859 and FAM101A rs7955740, were subsequently validated among a cohort of 113 patients. To date, clinical translation of SNPs as potential biomarkers for response is hampered by variability and poor reproducibility. Advances in large-scale genomic data handling may help overcome these limitations in future studies.

Tumour immune microenvironment

The anti-tumour effect of cytotoxic agents and radiotherapy may in part be related to their immunomodulatory properties. Cytotoxic chemotherapy activates anti-tumour immune responses by directly stimulating T-cell responses, inhibiting immunosuppressive cells, and inducing immunogenic cell death.[58] Radiotherapy enhances innate and adaptive immune signalling pathways in the local tumour environment, while also stimulating a systemic immunogenic response through circulating chemokines and cytokines.[59] Understanding the immunomodulatory effects of these therapies is imperative to designing novel treatment strategies.

Immunological factors associated with pathological response remain poorly understood, and involve a complex interplay between various T-cell subsets and the tumour microenvironment. Several series investigating TIL subset densities before and after neoadjuvant CRT for rectal cancer reported pretreatment TIL density is associated with a higher likelihood of tumour regression and pCR. Teng et al. found enhanced tumour regression among 62 patients with high pretreatment CD8+TILs, high CD4+TILs, and low Myeloid-Derived Suppressor Cells (MDSC),[60] while Yasuda et al. found that CD8+ TIL density was an independent prognostic factor for achieving a pCR among 48 patients.[61] Anitei et al. also observed favourable tumour downstaging with high CD3+ and CD8+ infiltration in pretreatment biopsies.[62] The Immunoscore (IS) was used to assess intratumoural immune response. This simple scoring system quantifies the density of cytotoxic and memory T cells (CD3/CD45RO, CD3/CD8, or CD8/CD45RO) in the core of the tumour and its invasive margin to provide a score ranging from 0 (low densities of both lymphocyte populations in both regions) to 4 (high densities in both regions).[63] The IS has internationally validated as an independent predictor of disease-specific survival in colorectal cancer (CRC), superior to the classical TNM staging system.[64]

The stroma, a critical component of the tumour framework, plays an increasingly recognized role in coordinating immune responses which appear to influence tumour regression. An inverse correlation between stromal Foxp3^{+} cell (Treg) density and pathological response has been observed following long-course neoadjuvant CRT suggesting immunosuppressive Tregs may represent a potential target for neoadjuvant immune-modulating therapy.[65] Evaluation of stromal and intraepithelial (IEL) TIL density in 93 patients undergoing neoadjuvant CRT for rectal cancer found that CD8+ stromal density increased after therapy and high pretreatment CD8/FOXP3 IEL ratio was a predictor of favourable tumour regression.[66]

Modern oncotherapeutics has focused on exploiting the potential synergy of conventional (chemotherapy, radiotherapy) and novel (monoclonal antibodies) treatments to enhance tumour immunogenicity. The programmed cell death 1(PD-1) pathway represents a promising target for cancer immunotherapy. PD-1, an inhibitory checkpoint, is expressed on activated T cells. Binding with its ligands PD-1 and PD-2 downregulates T-cell effector function, while blockade of this pathway with PD-1 inhibitors (e.g. nivolumab and pembrolizumab) reinvigorates suppressed T cells within the tumour microenvironment. A phase III trial demonstrated promising clinical efficacy with pembrolizumab in dMMR CRC.[67] Tumour cells may express PD-L1 as a mechanism of immune invasion. Theoretically, PD-L1 expression represents a logical predictive biomarker for response to anti-PD-1 or PD-L1 therapy; however, available data have been conflicting. Preclinical and clinical studies have demonstrated that radiotherapy induces upregulation of tumour cell PD-L1 expression in CRC, supporting the synergistic potential of combining radiotherapy and PD-1/PD-L1 pathway inhibition.[68,69] Several clinical trials are currently ongoing to assess whether combining conventional neoadjuvant CRT with PD-L1 (NCT03102047, NCT 03127007) or PD-1 (NCT02948348) inhibitors may improve pCR rates and tumour downstaging.

Conclusion

In the modern era of personalized care, the genetic signature of cancer has emerged as a promising potential aid to risk stratification and guide to surgical decision-making. Therapeutic algorithms tailored to the biomolecular signature of the tumour are needed to improve disease control, avoid the morbidity of futile treatments, and enhance quality of life and survivorship. Neoadjuvant chemoradiotherapy should be administered only when benefit is likely and, conversely, local or minimally invasive alternatives should be considered when biologically appropriate.

References

1. González I, Bauer PS, Chapman WC, et al. Clinicopathologic determinants of pathologic treatment response in neoadjuvant treated rectal adenocarcinoma. *Ann Diagn Pathol.* 2020;45:151452.
2. van der Sluis FJ, van Westreenen HL, van Etten B, van Leeuwen BL, de Bock GH. Pretreatment identification of patients likely to have pathologic complete response after neoadjuvant chemoradiotherapy for rectal cancer. *Int J Colorectal Dis.* 2018;33(2):149–57.
3. Huh JW, Kim HR, Kim YJ. Clinical prediction of pathological complete response after preoperative chemoradiotherapy for rectal cancer. *Dis Colon Rectum.* 2013;56(6):698–703.
4. Patel SV, Roxburgh CS, Vakiani E, et al. Distance to the anal verge is associated with pathologic complete response to neoadjuvant therapy in locally advanced rectal cancer. *J Surg Oncol.* 2016;114(5):637–41.

5. Wallin U, Rothenberger D, Lowry A, Luepker R, Mellgren A. CEA—a predictor for pathologic complete response after neoadjuvant therapy for rectal cancer. *Dis Colon Rectum.* 2013;56(7):859–68.
6. Huh JW, Yun SH, Kim SH, et al. Prognostic role of carcinoembryonic antigen level after preoperative chemoradiotherapy in patients with rectal cancer. *J Gastrointest Surg.* 2018;22(10):1772–8.
7. Han YD, Kim WR, Park SW, et al. Predictors of pathologic complete response in rectal cancer patients undergoing total mesorectal excision after preoperative chemoradiation. *Medicine (Baltimore).* 2015;94(45):e1971.
8. Huang CM, Huang CW, Ma CJ, et al. Predictive value of FOLFOX-based regimen, long interval, hemoglobin levels and clinical negative nodal status, and postchemoradiotherapy CEA levels for pathological complete response in patients with locally advanced rectal cancer after neoadjuvant chemoradiotherapy. *J Oncol.* 2020;2020:9437684.
9. Guinney J, Dienstmann R, Wang X, et al. The consensus molecular subtypes of colorectal cancer. *Nat Med.* 2015;21(11):1350–6.
10. Lynch HT, de la Chapelle A. Hereditary colorectal cancer. *N Engl J Med.* 2003;348(10):919–32.
11. Eriksson J, Amonkar M, Al-Jassar G, et al. Mismatch repair/microsatellite instability testing practices among us physicians treating patients with advanced/metastatic colorectal cancer. *J Clin Med.* 2019;8(4):558.
12. Malesci A, Laghi L, Bianchi P, et al. Reduced likelihood of metastases in patients with microsatellite-unstable colorectal cancer. *Clin Cancer Res.* 2007;13(13):3831–9.
13. Mohan HM, Ryan E, Balasubramanian I, et al. Microsatellite instability is associated with reduced disease specific survival in stage III colon cancer. *Eur J Surg Oncol.* 2016;42(11):1680–6.
14. Des Guetz G, Schischmanoff O, Nicolas P, Perret GY, Morere JF, Uzzan B. Does microsatellite instability predict the efficacy of adjuvant chemotherapy in colorectal cancer? A systematic review with meta-analysis. *Eur J Cancer.* 2009;45(10):1890–6.
15. Benatti P, Gafà R, Barana D, et al. Microsatellite instability and colorectal cancer prognosis. *Clin Cancer Res.* 2005;11(23):8332–40.
16. de Rosa N, Rodriguez-Bigas MA, Chang GJ, et al. DNA mismatch repair deficiency in rectal cancer: benchmarking its impact on prognosis, neoadjuvant response prediction, and clinical cancer genetics. *J Clin Oncol.* 2016;34(25):3039–46.
17. Hasan S, Renz P, Wegner RE, et al. Microsatellite instability (MSI) as an independent predictor of pathologic complete response (PCR) in locally advanced rectal cancer: a national cancer database (NCDB) analysis. *Ann Surg.* 2020;271(4):716–23.
18. Yan T, Seo Y, Kinsella TJ. Differential cellular responses to prolonged LDR-IR in MLH1-proficient and MLH1-deficient colorectal cancer HCT116 cells. *Clin Cancer Res.* 2009;15(22):6912–20.
19. Martin LM, Marples B, Coffey M, et al. DNA mismatch repair and the DNA damage response to ionizing radiation: making sense of apparently conflicting data. *Cancer Treat Rev.* 2010;36(7):518–27.
20. Kang H, O'Connell JB, Maggard MA, Sack J, Ko CY. A 10-year outcomes evaluation of mucinous and signet-ring cell carcinoma of the colon and rectum. *Dis Colon Rectum.* 2005;48(6):1161–8.
21. McCawley N, Clancy C, O'Neill BD, Deasy J, McNamara DA, Burke JP. Mucinous rectal adenocarcinoma is associated with a poor response to neoadjuvant chemoradiotherapy: a systematic review and meta-analysis. *Dis Colon Rectum.* 2016;59(12):1200–8.
22. Simha V, Kapoor R, Gupta R, Bahl A, Nada R. Mucinous adenocarcinoma of the rectum: a poor candidate for neo-adjuvant chemoradiation? *J Gastrointest Oncol.* 2014;5(4):276–9.

23. Kim MJ, Park JS, Park SI, et al. Accuracy in differentiation of mucinous and nonmucinous rectal carcinoma on MR imaging. *J Comput Assist Tomogr*. 2003;27(1):48–55.
24. Song GA, Deng G, Bell I, Kakar S, Sleisenger MH, Kim YS. Mucinous carcinomas of the colorectum have distinct molecular genetic characteristics. *Int J Oncol*. 2005;26(3):745–50.
25. Reynolds IS, Furney SJ, Kay EW, McNamara DA, Prehn JHM, Burke JP. Meta-analysis of the molecular associations of mucinous colorectal cancer. *Br J Surg*. 2019;106(6):682–91.
26. Zhang H, Evertsson S, Sun X. Clinicopathological and genetic characteristics of mucinous carcinomas in the colorectum. *Int J Oncol*. 1999;14(6):1057–61.
27. Maier P, Hartmann L, Wenz F, Herskind C. Cellular pathways in response to ionizing radiation and their targetability for tumor radiosensitization. *Int J Mol Sci*. 2016;17(1):102.
28. Hugen N, Verhoeven RH, Radema SA, et al. Prognosis and value of adjuvant chemotherapy in stage III mucinous colorectal carcinoma. *Ann Oncol*. 2013;24(11):2819–24.
29. Shin US, Yu CS, Kim JH, et al. Mucinous rectal cancer: effectiveness of preoperative chemoradiotherapy and prognosis. *Ann Surg Oncol*. 2011;18(8):2232–9.
30. Ueno H, Murphy J, Jass JR, Mochizuki H, Talbot IC. Tumour 'budding' as an index to estimate the potential of aggressiveness in rectal cancer. *Histopathology*. 2002;40(2):127–32.
31. Kevans D, Wang LM, Sheahan K, et al. Epithelial-mesenchymal transition (EMT) protein expression in a cohort of stage II colorectal cancer patients with characterized tumor budding and mismatch repair protein status. *Int J Surg Pathol*. 2011;19(6):751–60.
32. Rogers AC, Winter DC, Heeney A, et al. Systematic review and meta-analysis of the impact of tumour budding in colorectal cancer. *Br J Cancer*. 2016;115(7):831–40.
33. Rogers AC, Gibbons D, Hanly AM, et al. Prognostic significance of tumor budding in rectal cancer biopsies before neoadjuvant therapy. *Mod Pathol*. 2014;27(1):156–62.
34. Trotsyuk I, Sparschuh H, Müller AJ, et al. Tumor budding outperforms ypT and ypN classification in predicting outcome of rectal cancer after neoadjuvant chemoradiotherapy. *BMC Cancer*. 2019;19(1):1033.
35. Lugli A, Karamitopoulou E, Panayiotides I, et al. CD8+ lymphocytes/ tumour-budding index: an independent prognostic factor representing a 'pro-/anti-tumour' approach to tumour host interaction in colorectal cancer. *Br J Cancer*. 2009;101(8):1382–92.
36. Chang DZ, Kumar V, Ma Y, Li K, Kopetz S. Individualized therapies in colorectal cancer: KRAS as a marker for response to EGFR-targeted therapy. *J Hematol Oncol*. 2009;2:18.
37. Soulières D, Greer W, Magliocco AM, et al. KRAS mutation testing in the treatment of metastatic colorectal cancer with anti-EGFR therapies. *Curr Oncol*. 2010;17 Suppl 1:S31–40.
38. Clancy C, Burke JP, Coffey JC. KRAS mutation does not predict the efficacy of neo-adjuvant chemoradiotherapy in rectal cancer: a systematic review and meta-analysis. *Surg Oncol*. 2013;22(2):105–11.
39. Bengala C, Bettelli S, Bertolini F, et al. Prognostic role of EGFR gene copy number and KRAS mutation in patients with locally advanced rectal cancer treated with preoperative chemoradiotherapy. *Br J Cancer*. 2010;103(7):1019–24.
40. Chow OS, Kuk D, Keskin M, et al. KRAS and combined KRAS/TP53 mutations in locally advanced rectal cancer are independently associated with decreased response to neoadjuvant therapy. *Ann Surg Oncol*. 2016;23(8):2548–55.
41. Martellucci J, Alemanno G, Castiglione F, Bergamini C, Valeri A. Role of KRAS mutation as predictor of pathologic response after neoadjuvant chemoradiation therapy for rectal cancer. *Updates Surg*. 2015;67(1):47–53.

42. Duldulao MP, Lee W, Nelson RA, et al. Mutations in specific codons of the KRAS oncogene are associated with variable resistance to neoadjuvant chemoradiation therapy in patients with rectal adenocarcinoma. *Ann Surg Oncol.* 2013;20(7):2166–71.
43. Lopez-Crapez E, Bibeau F, Thézenas S, et al. p53 status and response to radiotherapy in rectal cancer: a prospective multilevel analysis. *Br J Cancer.* 2005;92(12):2114–21.
44. Jakob C, Liersch T, Meyer W, Becker H, Baretton GB, Aust DE. Predictive value of Ki67 and p53 in locally advanced rectal cancer: correlation with thymidylate synthase and histopathological tumor regression after neoadjuvant 5-FU-based chemoradiotherapy. *World J Gastroenterol.* 2008;14(7):1060–6.
45. Chen MB, Wu XY, Yu R, et al. P53 status as a predictive biomarker for patients receiving neoadjuvant radiation-based treatment: a meta-analysis in rectal cancer. *PLoS One.* 2012;7(9):e45388.
46. Williamson JS, Harris DA, Beynon J, Jenkins GJ. Review of the development of DNA methylation as a marker of response to neoadjuvant therapy and outcomes in rectal cancer. *Clin Epigenetics.* 2015;7:70.
47. Exner R, Pulverer W, Diem M, et al. Potential of DNA methylation in rectal cancer as diagnostic and prognostic biomarkers. *Br J Cancer.* 2015;113(7):1035–45.
48. Jass JR. Classification of colorectal cancer based on correlation of clinical, morphological and molecular features. *Histopathology.* 2007;50(1):113–30.
49. Sun W, Sun Y, Zhu M, et al. The role of plasma cell-free DNA detection in predicting preoperative chemoradiotherapy response in rectal cancer patients. *Oncol Rep.* 2014;31(3):1466–72.
50. Molinari C, Casadio V, Foca F, et al. Gene methylation in rectal cancer: predictive marker of response to chemoradiotherapy? *J Cell Physiol.* 2013;228(12):2343–9.
51. Gantt GA, Chen Y, Dejulius K, Mace AG, Barnholtz-Sloan J, Kalady MF. Gene expression profile is associated with chemoradiation resistance in rectal cancer. *Colorectal Dis.* 2014;16(1):57–66.
52. Gim J, Cho YB, Hong HK, et al. Predicting multi-class responses to preoperative chemoradiotherapy in rectal cancer patients. *Radiat Oncol.* 2016;11:50.
53. Guo Y, Cheng J, Ao L, et al. Discriminating cancer-related and cancer-unrelated chemoradiation-response genes for locally advanced rectal cancers. *Sci Rep.* 2016;6:36935.
54. Nelson B, Carter JV, Eichenberger MR, Netz U, Galandiuk S. Genetic polymorphisms in 5-Fluorouracil-related enzymes predict pathologic response after neoadjuvant chemoradiation for rectal cancer. *Surgery.* 2016;160(5):1326–32.
55. Yang YC, Wu GC, Jin L, et al. Association of thymidylate synthase polymorphisms with the tumor response to preoperative chemoradiotherapy in rectal cancer: a systematic review and meta-analysis. *Pharmacogenomics J.* 2017;17(3):265–73.
56. Ho-Pun-Cheung A, Assenat E, Bascoul-Mollevi C, et al. A large-scale candidate gene approach identifies SNPs in SOD2 and IL13 as predictive markers of response to preoperative chemoradiation in rectal cancer. *Pharmacogenomics J.* 2011;11(6):437–43.
57. Kim JC, Ha YJ, Roh SA, et al. Novel single-nucleotide polymorphism markers predictive of pathologic response to preoperative chemoradiation therapy in rectal cancer patients. *Int J Radiat Oncol Biol Phys.* 2013;86(2):350–7.
58. Bracci L, Schiavoni G, Sistigu A, Belardelli F. Immune-based mechanisms of cytotoxic chemotherapy: implications for the design of novel and rationale-based combined treatments against cancer. *Cell Death Differ.* 2014;21(1):15–25.
59. Chajon E, Castelli J, Marsiglia H, De Crevoisier R. The synergistic effect of radiotherapy and immunotherapy: a promising but not simple partnership. *Crit Rev Oncol Hematol.* 2017;111:124–32.

60. Teng F, Meng X, Kong L, et al. Tumor-infiltrating lymphocytes, forkhead box P3, programmed death ligand-1, and cytotoxic T lymphocyte-associated antigen-4 expressions before and after neoadjuvant chemoradiation in rectal cancer. *Transl Res.* 2015;166(6):721–32.e1.
61. Yasuda K, Nirei T, Sunami E, Nagawa H, Kitayama J. Density of CD4(+) and CD8(+) T lymphocytes in biopsy samples can be a predictor of pathological response to chemoradiotherapy (CRT) for rectal cancer. *Radiat Oncol.* 2011;6:49.
62. Anitei MG, Zeitoun G, Mlecnik B, et al. Prognostic and predictive values of the immunoscore in patients with rectal cancer. *Clin Cancer Res.* 2014;20(7):1891–9.
63. Galon J, Costes A, Sanchez-Cabo F, et al. Type, density, and location of immune cells within human colorectal tumors predict clinical outcome. *Science.* 2006;313(5795):1960–4.
64. Pagès F, Mlecnik B, Marliot F, et al. International validation of the consensus Immunoscore for the classification of colon cancer: a prognostic and accuracy study. *Lancet.* 2018;391(10135):2128–39.
65. McCoy MJ, Hemmings C, Miller TJ, et al. Low stromal Foxp3+ regulatory T-cell density is associated with complete response to neoadjuvant chemoradiotherapy in rectal cancer. *Br J Cancer.* 2015;113(12):1677–86.
66. Shinto E, Hase K, Hashiguchi Y, et al. CD8+ and FOXP3+ tumor-infiltrating T cells before and after chemoradiotherapy for rectal cancer. *Ann Surg Oncol.* 2014;21 Suppl 3:S414–21.
67. Le DT, Uram JN, Wang H, et al. PD-1 blockade in tumors with mismatch-repair deficiency. *N Engl J Med.* 2015;372(26):2509–20.
68. Deng L, Liang H, Burnette B, et al. Irradiation and anti-PD-L1 treatment synergistically promote antitumor immunity in mice. *J Clin Invest.* 2014;124(2):687–95.
69. Hecht M, Büttner-Herold M, Erlenbach-Wünsch K, et al. PD-L1 is upregulated by radiochemotherapy in rectal adenocarcinoma patients and associated with a favourable prognosis. *Eur J Cancer.* 2016;65:52–60.

Index

For the benefit of digital users, indexed terms that span two pages (e.g., 52–53) may, on occasion, appear on only one of those pages.

Note: Tables and figures are indicated by an italic *t* and *f* following the page number.